A390

P9-CJV-035

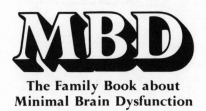

The Family Book about
Minimal Brain Dysfunction

Other Books by Richard A. Gardner

The Boys and Girls Book About Divorce
Dr. Gardner's Stories About the Real World, Vol. I
Dr. Gardner's Stories About the Real World, Vol. II
Dr. Gardner's Fairy Tales for Today's Children
Understanding Children: A Parent's Guide to Child Rearing
MBD: The Family Book About Minimal Brain Dysfunction
Psychotherapeutic Approaches to the Resistant Child
Psychotherapy with Children of Divorce
Dr. Gardner's Modern Fairy Tales
The Parents Book About Divorce
The Boys and Girls Book About One-Parent Families
The Objective Diagnosis of Minimal Brain Dysfunction
Dorothy and the Lizard of Oz
Dr. Gardner's Fables for Our Times
The Boys and Girls Book About Stepfamilies
Family Evaluation in Child Custody Litigation
Separation Anxiety Disorder: Psychodynamics and
    Psychotherapy
Child Custody Litigation: A Guide for Parents and Mental
    Health Professionals
The Psychotherapeutic Techniques of Richard A. Gardner

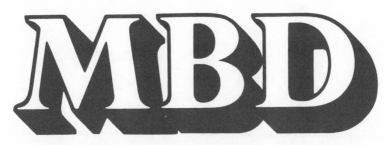

The Family Book about Minimal Brain Dysfunction

Part One: For Parents
Part Two: For Boys and Girls

RICHARD A. GARDNER, M.D.

Clinical Professor of Child Psychiatry
College of Physicians and Surgeons
Columbia University

ILLUSTRATED BY ALFRED LOWENHEIM

Jason Aronson Inc.
Northvale, New Jersey
London

TO LEE, ANDREW, NANCY, AND JULIE

This book is for the families of children with minimal brain dysfunction. The first part is for parents. It describes the physical and psychological aspects of the disorder, which parents should find useful in helping their child. The second part is designed to be read by children, preferably along with a parent.

Contents

Preface

Since the publication of my book, The Child's Book about Brain Injury several years ago, many things have happened in the field of minimal organic brain disorders in children. Although I was unhappy then about using the term *brain injury* (with its implication of the rarely applicable traumatic causative factor) in its title, it was the most commonly used term at the time. The far more accurate term, *minimal brain dysfunction,* is now sufficiently well-known to make its use possible in the title. The term *learning disability* has also become more commonly used to refer to this disorder (or to be more accurate, this group of disorders), and many have suggested that I use it. *Learning disability,* however, suggests to me the whole gamut of learning disorders, both psychogenic and organic in etiology. To use it to refer to the more specific class of disorders discussed in this book—manifestations of organic neurologic dysfunction—is misleading. The term *brain dysfunction* very specifically refers to the organic etiological factor, and so it is the one I prefer. Some of the

7

youngsters who read the first book were offended by the use of the word *Child* in the title and so I substituted the "safer" *Boys* and *Girls* in the subtitle.

There were so many requests for reprints and for permission to reprint my article, "Psychogenic Problems of Brain-Injured Children and their Parents" *(Journal of the American Academy of Child Psychiatry,* 7:471–491, 1968), and the response to the chapter on the treatment of children with minimal brain dysfunction in my recent book, *Therapeutic Communication with Children: The Mutual Storytelling Technique* (New York: Science House, Inc., 1971) was so gratifying that I decided to select material from those publications to include in this book as a special introductory section for parents. In this section I present an outline of the main organic and psychological manifestations of the disorder with some suggested approaches to the handling of the more common psychological problems. The second section, for children, is designed to be read by the child alone or along with a parent.

During the past few years we have witnessed a burgeoning of educational techniques that are of great importance for these children. Diagnostic methods for delineating more specifically its various manifestations and educational techniques specifically designed for teaching such children have been introduced at a staggering rate. In neurology, as well, there have been many advances in our appreciation of the wide variety of disorders that can manifest themselves as the syndrome of minimal brain dysfunction. These advances are not discussed in this book in detail. The primary purpose of the book is, through the guidance it offers, to relieve and avert some of the psychiatric difficulties that arise primarily from parental inexperience, naiveté, and misguidance. Although this book may also serve to mitigate and prevent some of the more severe difficulties that children with brain dysfunction may have, I am aware that, at best, it can play only a limited role in this regard, for such disturbances usually require more intensive approaches than just information and guidance.

8

Most children with brain dysfunction will not be able to read *Part Two* in one sitting. They could not possibly absorb all the information at once in a meaningful way. The Table of Contents is explicit enough for the child to select those topics that interest and concern him most. *I hope that the issues raised here will become points of departure for further discussions between parents and children.* Such conversations not only help resolve family problems, but also draw parents and children closer togther; and such mutual inquiry and cooperative discussion help to reduce the family difficulties that inevitably exist when a child has brain dysfunction.

Acknowledgments

My greatest debt of gratitude goes to the children with brain dysfunction who have taught me most directly and meaningfully what I present in this book. I wish to express my appreciation to Dr. Martha Denckla, Assistant Clinical Professor of Neurology, Columbia University, College of Physicians and Surgeons; Dr. Leo Sawitz, Director of Child Study, Tenafly Public Schools, Tenafly, N.J.; and Mrs. Carole Schwartz, Educational Therapist, Tenafly, N.J., for their thoughtful and useful comments. I am grateful to Mrs. Frances Dubner for her valuable editorial suggestions. Mr. Henry Marquit of the New York Association for Brain Injured Children was helpful in providing his organization's suggestions, cooperation, and support. Mrs. Linda Gould, my secretary, cheerfully undertook the task of typing the manuscript and its revisions. My wife Lee was most helpful in providing advice and recommendations derived from her own clinical experiences. Lastly, my deep gratitude goes to Dr. Jason Aronson, Jennifer Mellen, and Jane Lassner for their enthusiasm and dedication to the publication of this book.

11

Part One
For Parents

Introduction for Parents

When first learning of a book on brain dysfunction for children, the parent may wonder about the wisdom of presenting such a book to a child.

"Should I let my child know there is something wrong with his brain?"

"Wouldn't that upset him?"

These are typical responses of many parents who, with the best of intentions, feel that such a disclosure would be injurious to their children. In actual fact, an honest and open discussion with the child concerning his condition can be, in most instances, extremely helpful psychologically.

Imagine that you yourself were ill and that each time you asked your doctor what was wrong he became evasive or responded with platitudes. Sooner or later you would probably assume that you had some dreadful or incurable disease. Imagine, then, what it would be like to continually ask and to continually be put off and

15

ignored. For many, such responses produce extreme anxiety. It can be compared to the feelings you would have if you were lost at night in a forest or desert, aimlessly groping, not knowing in which direction to turn, and not knowing whether you will come out alive. As terrible as all this sounds, these are exactly the kinds of feelings children with brain dysfunction may have when they are kept in the dark about their condition.

The child's thinking may go like this: "They always tell me what's wrong when I have a sore throat or cold. If they don't tell me about this, it really must be bad; it must be terrible if they won't even talk about it."

The child with brain dysfunction usually knows that he is different. Other children read better, catch a ball more easily, or laugh at jokes that he cannot understand. Often he is in a special class; he may be going to a doctor; and others may make comments to him confirming their awareness of his difficulties. And yet no one—not his parents, teachers, relatives, or neighbors—may have told him exactly what is wrong. His condition is spoken about in whispers, behind his back.

Children are much more capable of accepting painful realities than is generally appreciated and are far less fragile in this regard than most parents realize. More difficult for them to handle (and this is true for adults as well) are the anxieties associated with ignorance and parental furtiveness, for then fantasy runs free and their worst anticipations are neither confirmed nor refuted. Half truths produce confusion and distrust, whereas truth, although painful, engenders trust and gives the child the security of knowing exactly what his condition is. He is then in a better position to handle his situation more effectively. It is not surprising, then, to see many of these children develop fears and insecurities that might have been prevented to some degree by the simple anxiety-alleviating device of making the unknown known.

Although fears and anxieties are the most common emotional difficulties, others can arise in this atmosphere of secrecy and

16

furtiveness. Often, parents do not tell their children that they have brain dysfunction because the parents believe that the condition is incurable and that there is no help. They feel that nothing can be gained by such a disclosure. However, most of these children *can* be helped, and the outlook is much better than most parents realize. To believe that the situation is hopeless gives a heavy, unnecessary burden to parents and child and undoubtedly plays a role in producing further anxieties and other emotional difficulties.

When a child learns that he can improve, that his defects are not total—but are isolated to certain areas—and that there are others with similar conditions who make satisfactory adjustments in the world, many of his emotional problems can often be alleviated.

I do not wish to give the impression that lack of knowledge about the problem is the only cause of emotional symptoms in these children. This is a common cause, but it is by no means the only one. It is, however, the problem that can often be helped by the child's reading a book such as this, either alone or with his parent(s).

It is safe to assume that the child with brain dysfunction is aware that he is different. He probably suffers from some anxieties and insecurities, although these may not be readily apparent. The child, therefore, if he can comprehend the book's contents, will most likely benefit from the information in it.

A few children may find portions of the material presented here anxiety-provoking but, in my experience, this has not usually been the case. On the contrary, most children have exhibited a deep and enthusiastic interest in this book. More often than not, the anxiety has been in the parents rather than in the child. The parent who decides beforehand that this book will upset his child may very well be depriving him of the opportunity to read what may be vitally helpful to him. Let your child be his own judge. Let his inner defenses be the final arbiters. The child who finds this material too painful will be the exception, but he will be able to protect himself by showing a lack of interest or by refusing to read

17

the book. At worst, he will experience mild, temporary anxiety, but he will not suffer any permanent psychological disability. Such disorders come about only through prolonged exposure to traumas and disturbing experiences. If your child seems hesitant to read the book, do not pressure him. Instead, tell him that he need not read the book if he does not want to and that he may have it again should he change his mind.

Since many children with brain dysfunction have difficulty concentrating over long periods of time, I suggest that this book be read in a number of short sittings, rather than all at once. The length of each sitting should be judged by the child's interest: once he shows signs of fatigue or disinterest, stop then and continue at another time or day. As you go along, discuss with the child any points that may not be clear.

It is my hope that the issues presented here will become points of departure for further discussions between you and your child. Such conversations will not only help resolve the problems under consideration, but they will draw you closer to your child— thereby reducing the likelihood of further psychological problems that can add to your child's difficulties.

The Basic Concept of
Minimal Brain Dysfunction

Most psychological disturbances of children such as fears, truancy, and frequent nightmares, are not associated with demonstrable physical, electrical, or chemical changes in the brain tissue. But in the group of disorders known as minimal brain dysfunction, such physical abnormalities of the brain are either demonstrable or strongly suspected.

Although their intelligence may be normal or even superior, children with this disorder often have significant difficulty in learning and in their social relationships. The exact percentage of children suffering with this disturbance is unknown. My own guess is that it is about three to five percent. However, not only is the number of such children increasing (as is to be expected in our burgeoning population), but the actual proportion of children who show this difficulty is also on the rise. This is not the false kind of statistical increase that comes with more general awareness of the disorder and more sensitive diagnostic techniques (although these factors

19

certainly contribute to the rising incidence being reported). Rather, it is the result of improved obstetrical and pediatric techniques. Children who only fifteen to twenty years ago would not have survived pregnancy and childbirth are now doing so—only to suffer the effects of their narrow escape from death.

Minimal brain dysfunction is seen in children whose mothers have suffered with a variety of difficulties. During pregnancy, these include excessive bleeding, nutritional deficiencies, infectious diseases such as German measles, and overexposure to radiation (including diagnostic X-rays). The disorder is more commonly seen in babies who were born prematurely, in first-borns (possibly related to their mothers' longer labors), when parts other than the head appear first, and when other mechanical difficulties are present during the birth process. Toxemia of pregnancy, excessive bleeding during delivery, umbilical cord complications (such as cord around the infant's neck), and Rh incompatibility have also been implicated as causes. After birth, the disorder can result from any of the infectious diseases that can damage the central nervous system, such as meningitis and encephalitis. It has also been associated with a group of diseases known as the "inborn errors of metabolism" of which phenylketonuria (PKU) is probably the most well known. These genetically determined biochemical derangements interfere with the normal metabolism of substances that are necessary for normal brain cell functioning. In less specific ways genetic factors also play a role in causing brain dysfunction. There are families in which the disorder seems to be transmitted genetically. Relatives on one or both sides of the child's family may have exhibited symptoms of minimal brain dysfunction during their childhood.

Seizures, even those that are only associated with fever, are not only a manifestation of brain dysfunction, but the seizure itself can bring about further neurological impairment. The physician's traditional advice—that mothers try to prevent these fever-associated seizures by rapidly giving anticonvulsant medication at the onset of fever—is inadequate, as children's fevers often

20

rise so rapidly that convulsions often cannot be avoided. Most pediatric neurologists are now recommending that children with such seizures regularly take anticonvulsant medication from the first seizure until they are four. They advise that at age four, attempts be made to wean the child gradually from the drug—which should be given again, of course, if the seizures recur. I have seen a number of children whose minimal brain dysfunction appears to have been the result of the failure to put them on such a preventive program.

There are many other diseases, agents, and predisposing factors that have been implicated as causes of minimal brain dysfunction. I have mentioned only the most common. However, in spite of the long list of possibilities, there are still many children in whom the cause is unknown. They are categorized as having minimal brain dysfunction because they show the same symptoms that are characteristic of the disorder.

The Primary Signs and Symptoms

Primary signs and symptoms are the immediate signs of the basic organic impairment. The secondary signs and symptoms are psychological in origin and represent the child's psychological reactions to his physical disability. The symptoms of minimal brain dysfunction are many and complicated, and only the most obvious and well-known manifestations are outlined here.

A lag in one or more of the developmental milestones is one of the most common signs. Your child may have been late in sitting, standing, walking, talking, and bowel and bladder training, or in several of these activities. He may have been late in developing language. Often speech may not be late in onset, but the child has difficulty in communicating properly with the speech he has. He may, for example, use the word *up* for *down,* or *upstairs* for *downstairs.* He may have trouble counting or naming colors when others his age are doing so. Some of the other deficits to be described may also be manifestations of developmental lag (slow maturation

22

of the central nervous system) rather than irreversible destruction of nerve tissue (which also may be present in some children with minimal brain dysfunction). For example, your child may persist in reversing letters that are mirror images beyond the age when most children no longer show such confusion. Some of the "soft neurological signs," which I shall describe, are also the result of developmental lag.

Marked and continuous hyperactivity, which has an aimless quality, is often present. The mother may recall that while she was pregnant, the child with brain dysfunction was more active than her other children and that during infancy he was so restless he did not cuddle. Colic may be another manifestation of your child's hyperactivity. After infancy, your child may be "hypertalkative" and even describe his thoughts as coming too fast. In many cases the hyperactivity may be so incessant that the child is even restless during sleep. Sometimes hyperactivity is caused by anxiety, but it then appears primarily in association with stress. The hyperactivity associated with brain dysfunction, as already mentioned, is practically continuous.

My experience has been that organic hyperactivity is *reduced* in more than half of these children by certain stimulants such as dextroamphetamine (Dexedrine) and methylphenidate (Ritalin). Similarly, the hyperactivity in such children may *increase* when attempts are made to reduce it with sedatives such as the barbiturates. These stimulants then can help your doctor make the diagnosis and can be of therapeutic value as well. But, it must be remembered that not all children with brain dysfunction will be sedated by these stimulants; some, like normal children, become more active. Also, a small percentage of normal children will react paradoxically to these stimulants and the barbiturates. When the stimulants do not successfully reduce the hyperactivity, one of the tranquilizers usually will. And reducing your child's hyperactivity enhances his receptivity to learning. He will not learn very much if he's fidgeting, jumping out of his seat, or running around the classroom most of the day. These stimulants, besides reducing hyperactivity, have an alerting effect, which helps concentration. In addition, they improve certain types of perception and learning in ways that are not yet completely understood. Usually, the hyperactivity in children with brain dysfunction decreases spontaneously by puberty, and then medication for this symptom is no longer necessary.

Distractability, or poor attention span, is another symptom of minimal brain dysfunction. Your child may have difficulty differentiating between important and unimportant stimuli, so he becomes easily diverted from the learning tasks at hand. For example, most children recognize that the teacher's words are more important than the sound made by a pencil dropped in the back of the classroom. These children do not make this differentiation. They may consider the dropped-pencil noise of equal, if not more, importance and rush to the back of the room to find out what's going on. Or they may consider their inner thoughts of equal importance to the teacher's word. They are then labeled "daydreamers."

The distractability may be visual. For example, your child may have little or no trouble reading a single word presented on a flash-card, but he may have great difficulty with the printed page, where the array of words distracts him from the one he is focusing upon. Small classes and homework done in a quiet room without siblings, television, and outside noises can be most useful. If you can provide extra home tutoring in a consistent way without becoming exasperated or angry, your child's learning progress can be enhanced. Try to use the same texts and learning materials that your child uses in school. A few short sessions of concentrated learning are better than one long one. Weekend and holiday tutoring is best in the morning, when your child is alert and not yet tired by physical activity. The aforementioned stimulants can also help this symptom.

Your child may have coordination problems. His handwriting may be poor; he may have trouble throwing a ball, riding a bicycle, or running without tripping. His poor copying of geometric figures may be the result of either coordination or perceptual problems—differentiating between the two may, at times, be difficult.

Children with minimal brain dysfunction often have perceptual problems, and these directly interfere with learning. Difficulty in perceiving things visually is the most common problem. This is not due to an impairment in refraction or gross acuity (Your child's eyesight might be 20/20.), but rather in fine visual discrimination. For example, your child's copies of geometric figures may reveal fragmentation, angulation, rotation, and other distortions. He may have trouble differentiating between letters and words that are mirror images of one another, such as: *b* and *d*, *on* and *no,* or *saw* and *was*. Such "reversals" are normal to a certain extent in the first grade (We are reminded of the proverbial: "Mind your p's and q's."), but in these children the problem persists longer and is more severe. They may have trouble with depth perception, spatial relations, and in differentiating foreground from background. This is demonstrated by the child's poor performance in the hidden-picture game, where he is asked to find the objects and animals that are partially concealed in a complex scene.

Auditory perceptual problems may also exist. Again, this is not in the area of auditory acuity, which is usually normal, but rather in fine auditory discrimination. For example, your child may have trouble discriminating between two words of similar but not identical sound such as *book* and *brook*. Auditory synthesis may be impaired—that is, when a word is spoken, but broken down into its phonic elements, your child may have difficulty fusing the parts to form a word he would ordinarily know. For example, he would not recognize *b—oo—t* to be *boot*. Auditory memory may be deficient. Your child may have trouble remembering what is read to him, but he will well remember that which he reads. When presented with a series of numbers, he can repeat fewer than other children his age. The ability to organize auditory stimuli into proper sequence may be impaired. For example, your child may not be able to accurately imitate rhythmic patterns of tapping. Dextroamphetamine can often help these visual- and auditory-perceptual impairments, thereby enhancing your child's learning ability.

Tactile perception may also be deficient. While his eyes are closed, your child may not be able to recognize letters marked out on his palm. He may not be able to differentiate between large and small coins placed in his hand.

Poor retention of what is learned is another common symptom of minimal brain dysfunction. This is characteristically erratic —there will be times when your child appears to have good retention, and other occasions when you will have the feeling that he has "a brain like a sieve." He may not only have difficulty remembering what he has learned in school but may also not learn from his errors —thereby repeating his mistakes, no matter how serious the consequences. Often the memory impairment is confined to a specific sensory modality. For example, his auditory memory may be deficient, while his visual and tactile memory are intact. Dextroamphetamine and methylphenidate can improve perception and retention in many children with minimal brain dysfunction.

Your child may have difficulty forming concepts and abstractions at an age when others are doing so. He therefore does not appreciate age-appropriate jokes and humor, has trouble with mathematics, and cannot understand the rules of games when he plays with other children. Such deficiencies may play a role in his becoming unpopular with other children.

Impulsivity is another problem often exhibited by children with minimal brain dysfunction. The child appears as if he has trouble "putting brakes" on his thoughts, feelings, and actions. This phenomenon probably contributes to the "catastrophic reaction" observed in younger children with this disorder. In this reaction to disturbing stimuli (the exact nature of which may not be known to the observer), the child exhibits a tantrum that does not have the angry element of the traditional temper tantrum but rather a quality of frustration, helplessness, and deep pain. Enuresis (bedwetting), which is probably more common in these children, is possibly another manifestation of poor impulse control. The older child may verbalize his frustration over not being able to control himself. His teacher finds him disruptive in the classroom: he calls out his thoughts and leaves his seat frequently. He is easy prey to bullies because he cannot refrain from responding to taunts and provocations in any but the most primitive manner. Tranquilizers and dextroamphetamine can often reduce this symptom.

Related to the impulsivity is repetition of speech often seen in these children. They repeat the same thing many times like a broken record. It is as if they were "hooked" on a certain word, phrase, or topic and cannot "unhook" themselves. Your child may persist in asking the same question until you are distraught.

Dominance of one side of the brain over the other, which determines right- or left-handedness and -footedness, may not have been strongly established. There may be crossed dominance: right-handedness and left-footedness, for example. Ambidexterity may also be present when dominance has not been strongly established.

So-called "soft neurological signs" are often present. These can be roughly classified in two groups. The first consists of subtle but definite physical signs of neurological impairment: minor coordination deficits, slightly hyper- or hypoactive reflexes, and minor muscle asymmetry, for example. The second group of "soft neurological signs" consists of those which represent lags in neurological development. For example, the grasping reflex (as opposed to voluntary grasping) is present at birth and normally disappears at sixteen to twenty-four weeks of age. A child of fifty weeks who still has a grasping reflex has an impairment of the nervous system. At sixty weeks, his fingers may no longer reflexly grasp when his palm is stroked—and so the sign is no longer present.

These neurological impairments, which are confirmation

27

of the syndrome's *organic* origin, do not necessarily show up in an electroencephalogram (EEG). Many parents ask for a "brain wave test" because they consider it to be the most sensitive indicator of the presence of the disorder. But the EEG is only abnormal in very specific types of neurological disorder. A child may exhibit significant brain dysfunction and still have a normal electroencephalogram. Accordingly, an EEG is of little diagnostic or therapeutic significance for the overwhelming majority of these children. It is only when diseases other than minimal brain dysfunction are suspected—diseases whose diagnosis and/or treatment may be aided by it—that the EEG should be obtained.

Finally, children with minimal brain dysfunction exhibit generally disruptive behavior for which there is no specific psychological term. They are called "bad" and told that they "just don't listen." They don't seem to be able to learn and follow the usual *right's* and *wrong's* and the *do's* and *dont's* as well as other children. Once again, dextroamphetamine and methylphenidate can sometimes dramatically change these children, and they may become "good" for the first time in their lives. They may show a response to reward, guidance, instruction, and threat that was never seen before—a boon to all who are involved with them.

As is true of many syndromes and diseases, no child exhibits all the signs and symptoms. Your child will manifest some, depending on the way in which his particular brain has been affected. The child who exhibits only one or two of the aforementioned symptoms —especially in mild degree—would not be designated as having brain dysfunction. It is only when a cluster of these symptoms is clearly present that the diagnosis is justified.

The Secondary Signs and Symptoms

In the past, some children with minimal brain dysfunction were considered to be suffering from purely psychological difficulties. There are, in fact, some who still hold the view that the total constellation of signs and symptoms that I have described is psychological in origin. Treating these children by traditional psychotherapeutic techniques has often proved futile, however, and their parents were burdened with guilt and unnecessary expense. In my opinion, the treatment of these children involves four approaches: (1) medication, (2) education, (3) parental guidance, and (4) psychotherapy (in that order).

Because so many of your child's signs and symptoms may be alleviated with medication, it is not fair to deprive the child of a trial. There are some parents who are reluctant to place their child on a drug regimen that may last for years. They fear the child may become addicted or that he will suffer significant side effects or toxic reactions. Even though dextroamphetamine, and some of the other stimulants used in the therapy of minimal brain dysfunction, can be addicting, I myself have never seen a child with minimal brain dysfunction become addicted to it. Generally, the drug can be discontinued at puberty, before youngsters who do become addicted start to use drugs. Others with considerable experience in this area agree with me that these children rarely become addicted to the medication that was prescribed in their childhood. I am not saying that the child with brain dysfunction is immune to becoming addicted. (In fact, as I will explain later, he may be more prone to becoming an addict than the normal child.) What I am saying is that psychological problems are the primary determinant of whether a child becomes addicted, not the administration of a drug for the treatment of a medical disorder. Also, the feared side effects are usually mild and are more than counterbalanced by the benefits the child obtains from the medication. Dangerous toxic reactions are rare with the stimulants and tranquilizers that are used to treat children with brain dysfunction (at the usually administered doses), and even these can usually be avoided by proper medical attention. I have never seen a child suffer anything more than a temporary unpleasant side effect from any of the drugs generally used for these children. And such reactions are easily alleviated with a smaller dose or discontinuation of the medication. The parent who will not allow his child to be placed on medication is being unduly cautious and depriving his child of an agent that has proved to be effective. Under the guise of protection he is doing the child a great disservice. Once the child has been properly medicated, he is more likely to benefit from the next step in his management: education.

Everything possible must be done to enhance your child's learning because many of his psychological problems are significantly related to his learning disability. In educating such children the exact nature and extent of the neurological impairment, especially in perceptual areas, must be determined. Attempts should be made to educate him primarily through his intact or better functioning sensory systems—just as the blind man learns to read tactily with Braille. In addition, there are special educational techniques that are designed to strengthen the defective areas. Educating children with brain dysfunction is an expanding field, and many useful devices and approaches have been developed in recent years.

Most children with minimal brain dysfunction develop secondary psychological difficulties. These often diminish as the primary neurological impairments improve through natural growth or education. Guidance and understanding on your part (of the type that I will present here) can also be helpful in alleviating these secondary psychological problems. Most children do not require any more than special medication, education, and parental guidance. In some, however, the secondary problems reach such a degree that psychotherapy is wise. Sometimes family problems contribute significantly to the child's psychological symptoms. Sometimes, in spite of the parents' deep interest, appropriate handling, and healthy involvement with the child, he still develops significant psychological difficulties. This should not be surprising when you realize that the disability can be so devastating that it colors the child's whole life. Wherever he goes, his difference from others may be obvious to all; he cannot escape his impairments; and he cannot run from his humiliations.

The common secondary psychological problems of children with minimal brain dysfunction cannot be adequately understood without considering their parents' problems as well. To make my presentation clear, therefore, I have divided further discussion into two sections: (1) the problems that may occur that primarily stem from the parents, and (2) those difficulties that, for the most part, arise in the child. The distinction is often artificial, however, because the symptoms of the child and those of his parents overlap. Each one's problems complement and contribute to the other's to such an extent that each symptom can best be understood as an attempt at resolution of, or adaptation to, a multiplicity of complex interacting forces in both child and parents.

The reactions of most parents can be separated into two types—acute, and chronic. In general, the acute adaptations are temporary and occur when the parents first learn of their child's brain dysfunction. The chronic adaptations may be extensions of the immediate reactions, or they may arise afterward. The distinction is important because the acute reactions have a good chance of clearing up either without treatment or with the kind of explanatory approach I present here, whereas the chronic reactions may become deeply entrenched and may require psychotherapy. In some cases, the distinction may be unclear or of little significance.

Your child's reactions do not easily differentiate between the acute and the chronic. The child has no acute reaction to learning of his disability; he grows up with it. Rather, it is a process of gradually realizing his impairment and then slowly developing neurotic—and sometimes psychotic—reactions. In my discussion of your child's signs and symptoms I will include both the explanatory approaches and some of the psychotherapeutic techniques I use when I work with a child with brain dysfunction.

ACUTE PARENTAL ADAPTIVE REACTIONS

The inappropriate acute psychological reactions by the parents of the neurologically impaired child are attempts to adapt to the child with brain dysfunction. This type of reaction, however, does not happen just because of the knowledge of the child's defect, but is partly determined by the parents' personalities.

THE DENIAL REACTION. A common reaction when some parents are first told the doctor's diagnosis is to deny it. Sometimes parents doubt the doctor's competence. The family may then embark upon a pilgrimage that can last for years, consulting one expert after another. Those who confirm the original diagnosis are also rejected. Their quest, of course, is for the physician who will say that nothing is wrong or that the child will outgrow his difficulties. They are looking for the doctor who will help them deny what they do not wish to see or hear.

Don't you become a "comparison shopper" of doctors. It is natural—and wise—to seek a second and even a third opinion. But if the doctors who see your child all agree, accept their diagnosis. During a "doctor-shopping" campaign, your child is not only deprived of valuable educational and therapeutic experiences, but any psychological problems—which might have been alleviated if the parents had accepted the diagnosis—may deepen. Furthermore, during this search for a "good" doctor, the child may infer the parental message: "We don't like you the way you are. We want you to be different. We'll find a doctor who'll tell us you are the way we want you to be." The devastating effect that such statements may have in lowering your child's self-esteem are elaborated on in the section devoted to the child's psychological problems.

There are some parents who deny the diagnosis by deciding that all behavorial problems are purely psychological in origin, and they may be given professional support for their position. To them, the idea that something is organically impaired implies permanence and incurability, whereas psychological disorders are considered amenable to—i.e., "curable" with—psychotherapy. Although it is certainly true that impairments manifested in the *severe* forms of organic brain dysfunction may remain throughout life and be relatively unaffected by any form of therapy, the milder types usually improve to some extent with the therapeutic approaches, that I will describe. Besides, purely psychological disorders are not so predictably amenable to therapy that one can be unequivocally optimistic about the outcome of treatment.

THE OVERPROTECTIVE REACTION. Another way of denying your child's illness in the early stages is to overprotect him. By keeping the child an infant, his parents seek not to expose the defects he will show as he matures, and they avoid confronting the painful reality. One insightful mother put it very well: "If your

33

child can't walk, then carry him. Then no one will know what's wrong with him." In addition, the parent might also be attempting to lessen the guilt he may feel over his child's illness (to be discussed later) by being overpermissive and indulgent.

Treating the child as an infant, of course, robs him of the opportunity to mature in areas in which he might be capable. This can only bring about even greater feelings of inadequacy than he might have had with the given defects. There are many other elements that contribute to parental overprotection. I mention here only those factors that relate to the child with brain dysfunction.

THE ANGER REACTION. Once a parent has accepted the diagnosis, a host of further reactions are common. Anger is one of the most frequent. You may think, "Why me?" "Why not my neighbor or the guy at work?" or "What a curse!" Such anger, which I consider to be a normal reaction in the early stages of acceptance, stems from the feelings of helplessness and frustration one usually feels with a child with minimal brain dysfunction. The anger reaction is abnormal, however, when it is prolonged and replaces positive, effective action. It will probably never disappear completely, but some parents direct their anger into socially useful channels. In their irritation with "neglectful and slipshod school systems," which fail to provide adequate facilities for their children, they may rise to the occasion and fight the "powers that be." Through such efforts, they may be instrumental in setting up schools and other facilities for the benefit of their own and other children with brain dysfunction. Community organizations for children with brain dysfunction not only serve their immediate purpose of improving the lot of these children, but are psychologically healthy and constructive outlets for many pent-up feelings the parents may have.

There are parents, however, who have great justification for anger. They have not denied their child's limitations. They have not sought an expert to tell them that nothing is wrong. Rather, they have been frustrated by the ignorance of the "experts" whose advice they have sought. Well-meaning physicians have told them not to worry, that the child will outgrow his "difficulty." Well-intentioned psychiatrists and psychologists have decided the cause of the disorder is purely psychological and may even have instituted treatment (at no small expense and time). Or, the child may have been misplaced in school—in a class for the retarded or emotionally disturbed, for example. The anger of these parents is understandable; but if they dwell on their misfortune or let their anger interfere with providing their child with proper professional attention and care, they only prolong their child's difficulties. As knowledge about this disorder becomes more widespread, such unfortunate occurrences will certainly become less frequent.

THE INAPPROPRIATE GUILT REACTION. Inappropriate guilt is a common reaction after learning of the child's illness. It may take the form of preoccupation with various transgressions and errors that might have brought about the illness. "It's all my fault. I didn't go to church enough." "God punished me for my sexual life before I was married." "Masturbation, that's what did it; it ruined my sperm."

Classical Freudian psychoanalytic theory proposes that guilt of this sort is often related to unconscious hostility toward the child and that his having the impairment is the "magical" fulfilment of those unconscious hostile wishes. Probably this classical formulation does apply in some cases. However, this guilt reaction is almost always present to a greater or lesser degree, and so the classical interpretation attributes exaggerated hostility to *just about all* parents of organically damaged children.

In my opinion, guilt of this sort is more often understood as a futile attempt to control an uncontrollable situation. The parent, by attributing the cause to himself, puts into his own hands the power to control what is otherwise uncontrollable. By making the illness his own fault, he implies that he could prevent its re-

35

currence by not practicing those transgressions that allegedly brought it about. This guilt, then, is a defense mechanism against anxiety over calamities to which we are all exposed and that are often impossible to prevent. I have occasionally seen references to this type of guilt mechanism in psychiatric publications; but it has not, I believe, been given the attention it deserves.

If the therapeutic approach to such parents tries to uncover unconscious hostility, they may become even more guilty and anxious. The therapist's directly denying the parent's responsibility is most often useless, because the parent must then face the helplessness that he cannot tolerate. But reactions like this are common. They show that such parents love their child and that they care and wish they could have prevented the illness in some way. Participating in a community organization for children with brain dysfunction can also help relieve this guilt. Working with these associations gives such parents a feeling of some control over the child's present and future situation and lessens the need to obtain this control through magical mechanisms such as inappropriate guilt. In addition, these activities are reparative and guilt-alleviating; that is, such action brings about the child's improvement, so there is less to be guilty about.

Another form of guilt that some parents have is related to the resentment that is almost always felt toward the neurologically impaired child. Many of these children *are* terrible burdens and may significantly disrupt their families. The frustrations and disappointments that their parents suffer are bound to result in angry reactions toward the child—reactions that may or may not be repressed, depending on how the parent deals with his anger. Some parents cannot believe that their anger is predictable and inevitable in such a situation, feel very guilty about it, and cannot accept it within themselves. Appreciating that mild to moderate resentment is normal can be helpful. Group discussions among parents of children with brain dysfunction may be even more effective in alleviating this form of guilt, because the parent witnesses for himself the hostile verbalizations of others and thereby feels less unique and loathsome.

THE BLAME REACTION. In guilt reactions, the individual blames himself. In the blame reaction, he considers someone else to be at fault. Like the guilt reaction, the blame reaction places responsibility in the hands of mankind and protects one against the feelings of helplessness that are common in parents of children with brain dysfunction.

When looking for someone to blame, the parent may select the doctor, who, being fallible, has defects, that now become elaborated upon. One doctor may become generalized to all doctors, who are then considered bunglers, incompetents, or charlatans. The doctor "at fault" may never even hear that he is to blame; but the child with brain dysfunction may never be able to forget it, so inculcated is it into him through his parents' complaints. Such an adaptation may undermine the child's faith in and respect for physicians. This may interfere with any therapeutic benefits he might otherwise derive from relationships with other doctors and therapists.

"WHAT TO TELL PEOPLE?" A common problem that arises in the early stages of accepting the diagnosis of minimal brain dysfunction is that of "what to tell people?" "People" here can be broken down into three groups: (1) your child, (2) his brothers and sisters, and (3) the world at large (the most important members of which are those "vicious, gossiping neighbors").

Regardless of the particular term that your doctor names the syndrome, the basic disorder is an organic disease of the brain; and you should try to impart this concept to your child. There is no term that, by itself, is anxiety-provoking to a child; but any term can become so if you, the parents, consider its use to be detrimental to him. I believe that you should give your child a simple and yet meaningful explanation of his disorder—taking into account his age and ability to understand. He should be told that a small part, or parts, of his brain is not working well and that as time goes on, as he grows, and if he works at it, things should improve. To make the explanation more meaningful, refer to your child's specific impairments. For example, "The part of your brain that helps you remember is weak. You have to work harder than other children to make things stick in your brain." The explanation should be concrete, because these children often have difficulties in conceptualizing. It is easier for your child to understand that things don't stick well in his brain than to appreciate that he has a poor memory.

Emphasize to your child that his impairment only means he cannot do *some* things as well as other children, to lessen the possibility that he will generalize and consider his isolated impairment evidence of total worthlessness. Your child was not born with an exaggerated reaction to any term; if he has one, he got it from others. If you take a more matter-of-fact attitude, so will your child. To avoid the truth or to couch explanations in euphemisms results in the child's thinking that his illness is far worse than brain dysfunction, that it is an illness too terrible to talk about. The anxieties this arouses may contribute to anxiety-alleviating symptoms, neurotic or even, sometimes, psychotic. In addition, such attitudes make the child distrustful of his parents, a situation that can have serious psychological consequences.

The way in which disclosure can, on occasion, dramatically alleviate such anxiety and defense mechanisms is illustrated by the following example:

Ben was a twelve-year-old boy known to have brain dysfunction since age five. At age nine, he became preoccupied with dinosaurs and collected books on the subject. The topic occupied a major portion of his conversation. At the same time, he became much more withdrawn and would spend hours on the floor clapping his hands or banging blocks together. He was referred to me because a diagnosis of schizophrenia had been added to that of brain dysfunction by the school psychologist, and the parents sought another professional opinion.

My clinical evaluation confirmed the psychologist's diagnosis. Ben was in a special class for children with brain dysfunction, cerebral palsy, and other disorders associated with impaired learning. Acting on the advice of physicians and teachers, however, Ben's parents had never told him what was wrong with him. His questions about this were always evaded, even though he was of normal intelligence and would have well understood reasonable explanations.

In the first interview, Ben drew a picture of a dinosaur and explained, "The dinosaur is the biggest animal that ever lived, but he was also the stupidest because he had such a very small brain. He was so big and clumsy he could destroy whole cities when he walked." Clearly, Ben considered himself big and clumsy with a small, stupid brain. The hostility expressed in the destruction of cities was found on further investigation to be related not only to the frustrations he suffered by being neurologically impaired, but also to the anger he felt toward his parents for their secretiveness about his disorder.

Ben's parents were advised to tell him about his brain dysfunction as directly and honestly as they could. They were reluctant to do this because of so many previous warnings to the contrary. I finally convinced them to follow my advice. I also told them I would continue to work with Ben, not only to discuss the diagnosis but also to help him with his reactions to the disclosure.

Two weeks and six sessions later, Ben was free from his dinosaur obsession, the withdrawal, and the hand-clapping and block-banging preoccupations. Although he still had some reactions not uncommon in the child with minimal brain dysfunction— feelings of inferiority, hypersensitivity to criticism, difficulties in interpersonal relationships—there was no evidence of the psychotic disturbance present for the three-year period prior to his first visit to me.

Although Ben's case is the most dramatic, I have seen many children whose neurotic, and even psychotic, symptoms were alleviated following such open discussion.

The general rule of openness and honesty should extend to your other children. They, too, will become anxious and suspicious of you if you avoid frank discussion. The ideal attitude that you can transmit to the siblings is one of acceptance of your child for what he is, sympathetic tolerance for his defects, and expectation that he will contribute to the household activities in the areas in which he is competent. If you and your other children look upon the child as a total cripple, feelings of inadequacy above and beyond what might be expected anyway may arise in him. A statement such as, "Don't give me that excuse. Just because you've got brain dysfunction and have trouble in school doesn't mean that you can't do your share of work around the house, just like your brothers and sisters," can be helpful in many ways. It prevents your child from using his brain disfunction as a maneuver to avoid responsibility for acts that he can perform; it enhances his self-esteem by your faith and expectation that he can perform well in certain areas; and it lessens the intensification of sibling rivalries that so often become exaggerated beyond their usual fierceness when the child becomes too much of a "privileged character." In regard to this possibility, statements to the other children such as, "Yes, we do have to give him extra attention in certain things, but in many ways he's treated the same as you. We'd do the same for you if you had brain dysfunction," can be helpful.

The problem of what to tell the neighbors is often a difficult one. The conflict seems to center on two issues: if you are open, you may be providing an honest atmosphere; but your child may be stigmatized and rejected by the neighbors and their children. If you do not tell the neighbors openly, your child is allegedly

40

being protected from their alienation. The latter course, however, communicates to your child that you are ashamed of what he is, and the deleterious effects of secretiveness that I mentioned before may result.

I favor the first course of action. All things considered, the wisest approach for you is one that would be similar to the one you would use if your child suffered from any other chronic illness. If you are matter-of-fact, there is a greater chance that the neighbors will be. However, even with such attitudes, there may be people who will react insensitively to your child. When such a situation arises, it should be treated like any other circumstance of a neighbor's reacting inappropriately to one's child. Tell your child that one occasionally meets people who have strange ideas and the neighbor should be looked upon as having a problem himself. In addition, it has been my experience that the neighbors usually become *more* tolerant when they are told what is wrong. The "bad boy" who should be taken in hand becomes the boy with brain dysfunction who cannot be held as responsible for his anti-social behavior.

CHRONIC PARENTAL ADAPTIVE REACTIONS

Although the reactions I am about to talk about may be prolongations of the acute phase, they may arise insidiously months, or even years, after the diagnosis has been made. These reactions are deeper and more complex, and they may require intensive psychotherapy or psychoanalysis to alleviate them.

THE MASOCHISTIC REACTION. I use the term *masochist* primarily to refer to someone who seeks out situations that bring about personal pain. It is the masochist's idea that the only way he can get love is to suffer. He does not consider himself worthy of attracting anyone who will treat him benevolently. He sees his choice as between being treated malevolently and being totally ignored. He selects pain as preferable to loneliness. He is too insecure to refuse the requests and demands made upon him, no matter how inappropriate or cruel. He feels that he must submit to the will of others or be abandoned. The masochist also measures the depth of his love by the pain he will suffer for the loved one. To the latter he essentially communicates, "I must love you very much if I am willing to suffer so much on your behalf."

The child with brain dysfunction may be utilized by his parents to further their masochistic gratification. The sicker the child is (or is kept), the greater the neurotic gratification of the masochistic parent. Such parents are blocked in following through with recommendations to help the child, even though they may pay lip service to such attempts and act as if they were trying.

Masochism can be used to express hostility. Although the masochist asks for help, he may unconsciously thwart the doctor or anyone else involved in the child's treatment and leave him frustrated and angry. Additional hostility can be expressed by making the doctor feel guilty: "After all this time, you haven't helped him a bit, Doctor." The doctor or therapist may fall into the masochist's trap by reacting with hostility and retaliation, thereby unwittingly helping the masochist add to his suffering. The child, too, can become the target of such a parent's hostility and guilt-provoking maneuvers: "Look how much I do for you, you ungrateful good-for-nothing child; you show no appreciation."

The martyr, in my opinion, is basically masochistic; and what I have said about the masochist holds for him as well. Both believe that the only way they can get love from people who are important to them is to suffer, but the martyr gains additional benefit by advertising his woes and misery. The martyr is saying essentially, "How noble I am to be able to endure what others cannot. People will certainly admire me when they see or hear of my courage in suffering." He attempts to enhance his self-esteem through exhibitionistic self-torture. The martyr may advertise his woes in order to elicit this sympathetic admiration, or he may suffer in silence, praising himself for his courage and strength in not crying out. But even when mute, he still communicates his agony non-verbally through such mechanisms as sighs and painful facial expressions. The martyr who publicizes his agony gains the esteem of those who are impressed by such maneuvers; the martyr who mutely enjoys his pain earns *additional* veneration from those who consider suffering in silence an added virtue. By his moaning, complaining, and appeals to pity, the martyr tends to evoke sympathetic comments and commiseration. Such reactions from those who are close to the martyr only serve to reinforce this behavior, much to the detriment of the child. Children of such parents often become guilt-ridden and come to loathe themselves for the pains they are led to believe they cause their parents. In addition, since children model themselves after their parents, they may grow up to be martyrs and masochists themselves.

THE OVERPROTECTIVE REACTION. The overprotective reaction, which was briefly mentioned earlier, often serves to help the parents deny the child's illness by preventing him from reaching that stage of maturity which would expose his defects. Children with minimal brain dysfunction are perfect subjects for parents who have strong overprotective needs derived from other sources. The overprotection can serve to deny the hostility, either conscious or unconscious, that the parent may feel toward the child; it can compensate for feelings of inadequacy about parenthood; and, of course, the more helpless the child is, or is made to be, the greater the opportunity to prove one's adequacy and "superadequacy" as a parent. A parent with low self-esteem and feelings of worthlessness may attain a feeling of being needed and wanted by deluding himself into believing that he is "all the child has in the world."

In many of these maneuvers, the neurotic behavior thrives on the child's helplessness, and unconscious mechanisms keep the parent from doing things to take the child out of his dependent, helpless state. Also, such overprotection deprives the child of the benefits of limits and structure, which these children need even more than the normal child. Without such structure the child feels unprotected and anxious and may develop neurotic symptoms to handle these reactions.

THE WITHDRAWAL REACTION. The child might be used to justify the parents' avoiding meaningful interpersonal contacts because of fear of intimacy. The mother who feels she has "nothing else to give others" becomes so taken up with ministering to her child's needs that she may be "too tired" for social and sexual relations with her husband. This may even extend to avoiding her responsibilities to the child's siblings.

Closely related is the mechanism of using the child to gratify hostile impulses toward others, for the withdrawals described above may entail the removal of gratification from others for the purpose of hostile expression. For example, the mother who may not be able to directly express resentments that she feels toward certain relatives may claim that she is so involved with her child that she has no time for them.

THE "DOCTOR-SHOPPING" REACTION. The doctor-shopping syndrome, which serves the denial of the diagnosis, does not always stop once the diagnosis is accepted. The quest now changes from attempting to find a physician who says nothing is wrong, to a search for a doctor who will provide the magical cure. Such parents often greet the newest physician with fawning flattery, praising him for his skill and deprecating the numerous doctors who have preceded him. It is the naive physician who is taken in by this and joins the parents in the delusion of his deification. The doctor will usually recognize that he is being bribed with flattery and idolatry in the service of the parents' need for a magical cure. He knows that, with such a come-on, "the handwriting is on the wall" and that the parents will ultimately throw him on the ever-growing heap of fallen idols as he proves himself to be unable to bring about the miracles he was deified to perform. His successor will hear *his* name added to the list of the maligned.

As their frustration grows, the parents become prey to every quack and charlatan who offers them a miraculous cure. The quicker and more prodigious the proclaimed cures, the more enthusiastic and worshipful the parents become. They then "spread the word" about the healer's powers, to bolster their hope and deny his defects, adding thereby more followers of the cult of the particular hero of the day.

After a succession of disillusionments, the parents usually develop attitudes of resentment, bitterness, and distrust toward even the most competent and dedicated of doctors. All this, of course, has a devastating effect upon the child's ability to profit from a relationship with any doctor or therapist. Since the child's reactions to the therapist so often mirror those of his parent, cycles of deification and subsequent iconoclasm make it extremely difficult for the child to establish a meaningful relationship with him.

The therapist does best for such parents by trying to prevent his deification at the outset. He should explain to the parents that he will do his utmost, but also that he has no power to grow nerve cells where they do not exist. He must try to interrupt the futile quest, confront the parents with the consequences of their behavior, assure them that he appreciates that they are trying to do the best they can for the child out of love for him, and explain that by their quest they are actually interfering with his progress. Furthermore, let me strongly emphasize that such shifting of therapists prevents a trusting relationship from forming, not only with those treating the child for his disorders, but with all other authority figures who are trying to be helpful to him. Lastly, the parents should be told that all doctors and therapists are fallible, that none can perform miracles, but that there are many good and devoted ones who can help their child. If this approach is successful, the wasteful pilgrimage may be interrupted long enough to make some progress.

Although these chronic adaptive reactions may require psychotherapy or psychoanalysis to alleviate them, the therapeutic value of the community organization for children with brain dysfunction cannot be overemphasized. These groups are comprised primarily of parents and children with brain dysfunction, but they attract professionals and interested non-parents as well. They provide a wealth of information and services for such parents and are active in forming schools, special classes, and recreational programs for these children. They are often the lobbyists who get bills passed, money allocated, funds raised, buildings built, and teachers trained to teach their children. The milieu is constructive and creative. The parents' search for magical cures and possible bitter preoccupation with their lot in life is replaced by constructive action. Further, these groups can provide them with hope through positive action, a greater feeling of self-worth, and a feeling of camaraderie with other parents. Seeing others with similar problems can help them feel less depressed about their own difficulties. The groups also provide opportunities for the child to meet other children with brain dysfunction, the value of which will be discussed in the next section.

ADAPTIVE REACTIONS IN THE CHILD

THE FEAR REACTION. It is reasonable to expect that the child with brain dysfunction, ill-equipped as he is to cope with the world, will fear venturing forth into it. He is exposed to many frustrations and humiliations to which the normal child is not. He may not run as well, get the point of a game as quickly, read as well as others in his class, or perform as well as his friends in a host of other activities. He fears each new undertaking for the disappointment it may bring him. He tends to generalize and may foresee failure even in areas in which he is capable. Such fears can be reduced in a number of ways. Helping your child realize his areas of capability so he can avoid what he is intrinsically poor in, while participating in activities of competence, can be very helpful. Also, if he can improve through training, treatment, and growth, he will experience less fear of tasks in his deficient areas. Early educational experiences can also give these children the "head start" they so sorely need.

If you are an overly permissive parent, you may increase your child's fears. All children need the reassurance of parental guidance and control. Deprived of this, they become fearful, anxious, and insecure. The child with brain dysfunction needs much more supervision and regulation than the average child. Without these controls, he not only fears, but he may suffer guilt for what he does when uncontrolled. An orderly, predictable environment with appropriate restraints can be beneficial in reducing your child's fears.

If these fears have been compounded by his ignorance about his disorder, simple, direct discussion, as I have shown, can help lessen them.

THE WITHDRAWAL REACTION. There are various maneuvers that your child can use to avoid fears, humiliations, and rejections. The withdrawal reaction is one of the more common. The world of reality becomes too threatening; isolation and reversion to inner fantasy become more gratifying. In extreme situations, hallucinations may result. It is important to note here that in the psychotic without brain dysfunction the withdrawal is often based on delusional ideas about the world of reality. In the child with brain dysfunction, there is often more harshness in the reality from which he is withdrawing. Because it is based on reality, this type of psychotic reaction is easier to change. The case of Ben, the twelve-year-old boy who was psychotically obsessed with dinosaurs, is a case in point. In some children with brain dysfunction, however, the psychotic symptoms are an intrinsic part of the organic brain dysfunction syndrome; and these cases are most resistant to treatment.

The child's withdrawal may result in his failing to acquire skills that he might otherwise have been quite capable of learning. He becomes more inexperienced and naive about the world than his deficiencies would make him.

To the degree that you can make his environment less threatening and more inviting, you can reduce the chances that your child will withdraw. Placing the child in a special class with others with similar difficulties can be of great help. In such an environment, he feels more acceptable and is less subject to exclusion and embarrassment. Social and recreational groups for children with brain dysfunction serve a similar purpose.

THE REGRESSIVE REACTION. Another reaction that sometimes occurs is that of regression to levels of behavior even more immature or infantile than you might expect from your child's degree of impairment. The most common regressive manifestations are enuresis, rocking, baby talk, whining, silliness, clinging, temper tantrums, thumb-sucking, and balking at assuming age-appropriate responsibilities, such as dressing, making one's bed, and doing chores. By regressing, your child is protected from the embarrassments and rejections he might encounter if he were to attempt to function at a higher level. As previously mentioned, the overprotective mother may encourage this reaction.

Parental indulgence and participation is sometimes present when regressive symptoms exist. Often this is very subtle. For example, the parent might point out all the child's homework errors so that he can get a good grade. The parent may think he is helping him, but the child is thereby deprived of the mild anxiety over failure that is an important impetus to learning. The child's neurological impairment may be used as the parents' rationalization for allowing a perpetuation of the regressive symptoms.

In my sessions with these children I often point out to them that their regressive symptoms may be contributing to their alienation from peers by saying, for example, "When you get silly and use baby talk the other children don't want to play with you." I also confront the child with his regressive symptoms when he exhibits them to me, and I communicate as well my emotional reactions: "If you're going to act so silly, I'm not going to continue playing this game with you. It's no fun for me when you don't play seriously. And I know you can. I think this is one of the reasons why some of the children don't like playing with you." Most children can exert some conscious control over these symptoms, in spite of unconscious psychological factors that may contribute to them.

NEUROTIC UTILIZATION OF THE ORGANIC SYMPTOM. Some children with brain dysfunction will use the disorder to rationalize non-action in areas of competence. They may say, "I have brain dysfunction, so I can't do anything." The answer to this, of course, should be, "Yes, you have brain dysfunction; and it is true that there are some things that you cannot do as well as others, but that doesn't mean you can't do anything." They may tend to generalize and interpret their isolated defects as meaning that they are totally worthless. The child might say, "I'm just no good; I can't read." A parent might reply, "There is no question that it's harder for you to learn to read; however, there are many things you do and say that make me happy to be with you and have you as a child."

PERSEVERATION. Although perseveration is generally considered a direct manifestation of the neurological deficit, it also has, in my opinion, significant psychological elements. It can be used to gain attention. By repeating the same questions, the child prolongs a conversation and thereby avoids the dreaded isolation that is often his lot. This is not to say that such repetitions are not related to the child's inability to understand or retain the offered answer; but often the issue is one in which the child has demonstrated understanding. I encourage parents to stop the discussion after a few rounds and to express their reactions to it: "Look, this is getting on my nerves. I've answered that question four times. That's enough. Let's talk about something else." I suggest that the parents not only provide the new topic but also start discussing it in order to divert the child. If he still persists, I recommend that they tell the child that they will not respond to his further comments on that subject. They must then strictly carry out their warning.

Sometimes the perseverated issue is one that has important psychological significance that might not be immediately apparent from the topic the child is discussing. Early in treatment, a child patient of mine repetitiously complained of pain deep inside his "tushy" as well as eye pain. He also sniffed many foods before eating them and hesitated to eat those that he considered foul. I considered these preoccupations to show his feelings of self-loathing, related to his awareness of his deficits. Obnoxious material within him (his feces) is causing him trouble (pain inside his rectum); he doesn't have to add to his difficulties by ingesting further objectionable material such as malodorous food. His eye pain probably symbolized his awareness of his perceptual impairment; that is, he wasn't "seeing things right." His mother was advised to state simply that there was nothing wrong with his tushy, eyes, and the food he was eating and to discuss it no further. I, too, refused to engage in similar conversations. Focus on these particular symptoms would have only served to entrench them. I believed that with enhanced competence gained through education, medication, and psychotherapy, he would feel better about himself and these preoccupations would lessen—and this is what ultimately happened.

Sometimes—and this is especially true of younger children with brain dysfunction—the perseveration is related to a desire for further reinforcement of a previously rewarded response. For example, when the child is asked to count, the conversation may go like this:

Child: One.
Parent: Right, keep going.

Child: Two.
Parent: Good!
Child: Three.
Parent: Very good!
Child: Three.
Parent: Yes. Go on. What comes after three?
Child: Three.
Parent: Let's start again.
Child: One, two, three, three, three——

The child here does not know how to count past three. Since three has been reinforced by the parent's enthusiastic "Good!", he repeats it. He wants more compliments. He is similar to the child who tells a joke, gets a laugh, and then repeats the joke to enjoy once again the favorable response from those around him.

THE CLOWNING REACTION. Clowning is another common reaction. The child with minimal brain dysfunction is referred to as a clown or freak, and he responds by playing the role to the extreme. It is as if he were saying, "They call me a freak; it's not because I am one, but it's because I *have chosen to be one.* To prove it, I'll act like one. See, I can turn it on at will." The proof here, of course, is specious because, although he can turn it on at will, he cannot turn it off to the degree that he will not be labelled an "oddball." Dr. Leon Eisenberg of the Harvard Medical School puts it well: "Having been ridiculed when laughter was the very opposite of what they sought, they maintain the fiction that they are play-acting and seek the notoriety they fear they cannot escape."

In working with children who utilize this reaction, I try to get them to appreciate that although they may enjoy some temporary attention by their antics, those who laugh at them are not truly their friends—they do not invite the clowner to their parties, and they do not seek him out. When the child exhibits his silliness in a session with me, I do not encourage it with laughter but

51

rather react coldly to it and respond with comments such as "It's behavior like that that makes children not want to play with you" or "To me, you're no fun when you act that way. Enough of that baby stuff." I then try to encourage the child to involve himself in more mature activities.

IMPULSIVITY. Although the impulsivity of the child with brain dysfunction has an organic basis, there may be psychological contributions as well. If the child has been overprotected, the symptom may have been indulged. Anxiety increases impulsivity in most children whether or not they have brain dysfunction. The impulsive child may be singled out for bullying because the bully quickly sees that the child's inability to react with calm and restraint makes him predictably susceptible to taunts.

Most impulsive children can exert some conscious control over their outbursts—regardless of the factors, both organic and psychological, that may be contributing to their symptom. One can help such a child learn to inhibit himself. For example, a child in treatment often reacted with tears and effusive self-denigration whenever he lost a game. During a game of checkers, as I was about to make a double jump, I said, "I'm going to make a move now that might upset you. Let me see if you can hold yourself back from screaming out and calling yourself names." When the child did exhibit self-restraint, I complimented him. Helping the child to realize the detrimental consequences of his impulsivity can also help motivate him to restrain himself. I might say, for example, "Those boys pick on you because they know that you won't ignore them when they tease you. When you stop crying and screaming back, they'll stop teasing you because then it won't be any fun for them anymore."

REACTIONS TO THE LEARNING IMPAIRMENT. Some children with brain dysfunction are exquisitely sensitive to their deficits. Such insight is a mixed blessing. On the one hand, it may serve to motivate

52

the child to improve, while on the other hand it may enhance his psychic pain. Such children have a strong tendency toward self-deprecation. They also tend to generalize and consider their isolated defects to be proof that they are totally worthless as human beings.

As I have mentioned, it is important for you to impart the notion that only one small part of the brain is affected—the part that has to do with learning. You must repeatedly tell your child that the rest of him works fine, that just because one small part of him is not working well does not mean that he is completely worthless, and that it takes him longer to learn things and he has to work harder to do so. The point that no one is perfect and that everyone makes mistakes and has defects must be repeated many times over. Often, I will comment on my own deficiencies and errors as they occur in the course of my interchanges with the child. For example, if I cannot hear the child (I do have a hearing deficit), I might say, "Please speak a little louder. The nerves inside my ears don't work too well, and I have a little trouble hearing. Just as you have to work harder to learn, I have to work harder to hear." Or, when playing checkers, I might remark, "Gee, I missed that one. I'd better pay more attention to the game."

The child's feelings of shame over his learning impairments can be lessened if he is placed in a class with children with similar problems. When a school requests my opinion regarding class placement, I give this consideration highest priority. Some schools prefer to place children with brain dysfunction in normal classes and only take the child out of the classroom for special instruction. Although this plan may be satisfactory for children with *minimal* brain dysfunction, those with more severe dysfunction are usually mortified by such an arrangement. With it they not only must face the painful comparison with normal peers throughout most of the day; but in addition, when they are singled out to leave the room for special instruction, they suffer further humiliation.

THE ANGER REACTION. There are many reasons why anger is common in children with minimal brain dysfunction. There is much that frustrates them—things that continue to frustrate them in spite of their strongest efforts. They are rejected by peers for reasons that they are often ill-equipped to understand. Their parents may prefer their normal siblings. (I have known a number of parents who consciously or unconsciously omit mentioning their children with brain dysfunction when they discuss their families.) Their poor impulse control often prevents them from holding back their anger at the right times—thereby compounding their difficulties and providing them with another reason to be angry.

These children may directly express their anger, but more often they discharge it by means of neurotic (and sometimes, psychotic) mechanisms. The anger and the accompanying neurotic symptoms can only be lessened if the basic impairments are reduced or alleviated by education, medication, and psychotherapy.

THE LOW SELF-ESTEEM REACTION. The problem of low self-esteem is almost universal in children with brain dysfunction. As with most psychological symptoms, the roots are complex.

Although many factors contribute to the formation of psychological symptoms, they all contain attempts to compensate for low self-esteem. And while neurotic symptoms are formed to enhance feelings of adequacy, they usually result in lowering self-esteem even further. For example, the unpopular boy who lies to his peers and describes interesting and unusual exploits may enjoy more ego-enhancing attention at first; but as soon as his peers learn of his lies (and they inevitably do), he suffers more rejection than when he was unpopular but truthful. In addition, even before his friends suspect his lies, he has compromised his own dignity by lying. He is inwardly embarrassed about what he is doing, and this in itself reduces the ego-enhancement he had hoped to achieve. The class clown is laughed at but not liked by most of his schoolmates. He deludes himself into thinking that their enjoyment of his antics reflects respect; and if he is rejected in other areas, he may respond with even more harebrained escapades, which further alienate his peers. The child who buys friends with candy and money may experience temporary relief from his loneliness and its associated feelings of worthlessness, but he inwardly knows that his friendships are not true, that they are dependent upon continual bribery, and that he is being exploited. Accordingly, he feels even more inadequate than before. In short, such symptoms are, in part, misguided attempts to bolster a lagging self-esteem. What begins as a maneuver to enhance his feelings of self-worth ends up lowering it. This, in turn, may stimulate further utilization of the maneuver, resulting in an even greater loss of self-respect.

A young child, having no guidelines of his own, develops his self-image by what the psychiatrist Harry Stack Sullivan called "reflected appraisals." That is, the young child's concept of himself is derived essentially from his parents' opinion of him. It is only later, when he makes friends, enters other homes, and goes to school that new criteria for his self-worth are introduced. Modifications can then be made to alter distortions that may have come from the parents. In the healthy development of a child, two main processes take place: (1) increased experience and further modifications result in greater accuracy and reality of the self-image; and (2) the reliance on the environment decreases and that on the deeply formed inner convictions increases, so that a child's self-esteem is determined less by a changing environment and more by the tried and tested *inner* repertoire of criteria for deciding self-worth.

So deep and lasting, however, is this earlier "reflected appraisal" that a child whose parents despise him may never be able to gain a full feeling of self-worth. As a result, he may spend his life futilely using a variety of neurotic and even psychotic mechanisms to bolster his low self-esteem.

A young child lives by this dictum: I am what significant figures say I am. A three-year-old child may run to his mother crying, "Johnny called me stupid." The mother replies, "You're not stupid. He's silly," and the child stops crying. Hopefully, as he grows older, he will consider as well his own inner repertoire of criteria for self-worth—what *he* thinks of himself. Failure to do this leaves him at the mercy of all those who might criticize him. Since he can never be completely acceptable to everyone, he must sooner or later be exposed to disapproval. But accepting all criticism as valid can only result in his chronically detesting himself.

It is the job of parents and therapists to help the child with minimal brain dysfunction appreciate that he is not necessarily what others around him consider him to be. They must help the child enrich his set of criteria for judging his self-worth. They must help the child look *to his own opinions* as well as to those of *others outside his home.* The child must learn to consider with receptivity, but not with gullibility, the opinions of his parents and to accept what is reasonable and reject what is not. He must be helped to see his parents' distortions and their fallibility. The mother who says, "Your father doesn't think too much of you because you aren't very good in sports. To your father, sports are the most important thing in the world. There are many others who don't think that any single thing, like sports, is all that important, and they don't put down someone just because he isn't good at sports," is making a healthy statement. Her husband may consider her disloyal, but she has an obligation to her child, as well.

Feelings of competence must ultimately be based on some realistic attribute or skill. The two-year-old child who builds a tower of blocks beams over his accomplishment. His sense of mastery is ego-enhancing. The mother who says, "What a beautiful tower you've built!" directs her compliment to the product of the child's labors and raises his feelings of self-worth, increasing the likelihood that he will build again. In contrast, the mother who responds, "You're going to be a great builder someday and we'll all be proud of you; the family will be famous," uses the child's accomplishments for her own self-aggrandizement, lessens his pleasure and feelings of competence, and makes it less likely that he will derive ego-enhancing gratifications from building.

A common way in which parents contribute to a child's feeling of low self-esteem is by disparaging those who are successful. When the child does not compete successfully, he is told that others' rewards are undeserved, that they are due to good luck, or that they are the result of special favors and influences. The child's own inadequacies, which may indeed have contributed to his poor standing, are not even considered.

Compliments that are not related to any concrete accomplishments can be ego-debasing: "What a fine boy," or "Aren't you a nice girl," makes many children squirm. They sense that they are being "buttered up," and they are insulted as well because the comment implies that the speaker thinks they are stupid enough to be so taken in. But, "What a good cake you baked," or "Great, a home run," makes a child stand a few inches taller. This principle is well demonstrated by the adolescent who takes drugs. He does so, in part, to desensitize himself to the massive feelings of self-loathing he suffers because he has no area of competence or skill. To try to wean him from the drug without providing him with some training program in which he can gain a sense of proficiency and mastery is futile. Without proficiency in genuine skills, feelings of competence can at best be unstable. The child must, however, be discouraged from pursuits in which he has demonstrated particular ineptitude. For example, the child with minimal brain dysfunction, with a coordination defect, would suffer deep humiliation in a sports-oriented summer camp.

Feeling genuinely needed is another element that contributes to a child's sense of self-respect. One of the criteria I use to determine if a seriously depressed person is suicidal is whether he has the deep conviction that no one in the whole world would miss him if he were dead. Although children are dependent and need their parents far more than their parents need them, the child must still feel that his absence would be painful to his parents if he is to have a healthy feeling of self-esteem. (The healthy child in a loving home doesn't think about his parents' reactions to his absence, whereas this is often a source of concern to the deprived child.) The younger child feels elated over the fact that he can make others laugh. The child who helps mother set the table or helps father change an automobile tire glows with the feeling that he is an important and contributing member of the family team.

A cause of low self-respect for many children is the notion that they are the only ones who have the "terrible" thoughts and feelings that they harbor within them. Parents often confirm such suspicions and deepen the child's detestation of himself. The parent's reassurance that not only does he know many children with similar thoughts and feelings, but that he also has had, or still has, the same kinds of ideas and emotional reactions can help lessen the child's low self-respect.

Inhibition in asserting oneself is another source of low self-esteem. The child who is smouldering with pent-up hostilities over not having stood up for his rights has little respect for himself. He derogates himself because of his passivity, and his pent-up anger in itself prevents a feeling of self-satisfaction. Parents' encouraging the child to assert himself, to not allow himself to be taken advantage of, and to appropriately express his resentment can help alleviate such feelings of inadequacy. Neurotic factors notwithstanding, revenge *is* sweet. Winning a well-fought battle also enhances one's feeling of competence.

Although depression, in the adult sense, is not too common in childhood, one aspect of depression that is seen is the turning inward of hostility, with associated self deprecation. Such children, like their adult counterparts, are inhibited in openly expressing their resentments. They turn their anger inward against themselves (a safer target), and their self-flagellation and self-disparagement result in significantly lowering their self-esteem. The wise parent helps the child direct his hostility toward the appropriate source so that the irritations that are engendering the anger can be more effectively dealt with.

When a patient tells me, "I feel lousy about myself," I generally ask, "Are you doing anything that would make anyone feel lousy about himself were he doing the same thing?" Often, after some thought, I get an affirmative answer. The child may be cheating on tests, stealing, or lying excessively. If he has anything approaching a normal conscience, he will feel guilty about these acts. Intrinsic to guilt is self-loathing: "What a terrible person I am for doing all these horrible things." The child in such a situation might be told, "As long as you do those things you're going to find that you'll feel lousy about yourself. I think you'll see that if and when you can stop, you'll feel better about yourself." Although the proverbial advice, "Virtue is its own reward," may seem trite, it is most valid.

A child who is a perfectionist is unable to live up to the unrealistically high standards he sets for himself. He is therefore never satisfied with his performance and suffers from chronic feelings of inadequacy. Comments such as these may be helpful: "As long as you think that any grade below A is unacceptable, you'll feel lousy about yourself," or "As long as you feel you have to be the best basketball player in every game in order to be acceptable, you'll feel terrible about yourself."

The parent who, under the guise of helping his child with his homework, actually does it for him or points out his mistakes so that the child can hand in perfect papers is seriously undermining the child's self-confidence. The child cannot possibly enjoy a feeling of mastery if he has not indeed "mastered" his subject. The father who makes the models for his child so that they "look better" is sabotaging the child's attempt to gain a feeling of self-confidence. These are but two examples of the overprotective parent–overdependent child syndrome. Such children become psychologically paralyzed; they are incapable of performing up to their age levels in many areas; they cannot help but compare themselves unfavorably with their peers; and they inevitably suffer massive feelings of inadequacy.

Your child with brain dysfunction cannot do some things as well as other children, but he is undoubtedly aware of this without your pointing it out to him. He will feel much better about his accomplishments, however, if you praise him, do not exaggerate their worth, and let him do his work by himself as much as possible.

Whereas I recognize that a healthy parent will not completely accept *everything* in the child with brain dysfunction, neither will the loving parent generalize and consider the child totally worthless because of certain defects. The child's self-image will, in part, mirror that of the parents; and he will generalize to the extent that they do. The parents who doctor-shop, hide the diagnosis from the child, family, and neighbors, and overprotect or deny the illness all share the basic attitude of not accepting the child for what he is. For example, parents with inordinately high academic standards, who equate education and intelligence with happiness, will not accept a child who might become a perfectly adequate tradesman or craftsman and, in his own way, have a rewarding life. Such parents are, in effect, saying to the child, "You are a totally worthless person because you aren't smart in school." Parents who put great emphasis on sports or physical prowess may reject the poorly coordinated child whose chances of academic gratification and competence in many other areas are good. These parents, too, may consider their child totally worthless because of their own need to mold him into a preconceived pattern of what a worthwhile child should be like.

The child who is rejected because of his brain syndrome must be helped to appreciate that this does not mean that he is unlovable. Because someone rejects him does not make him rejectable. He must be helped to appreciate that he can still get affection from others—both at present and in the future. Meaningful involvements with peers as well as with adults can provide the child with substitutive gratifications to compensate him for the rejections he suffers. With peers this is more likely to occur if they also have brain dysfunction, and every effort should be made to place the child in situations where he is most likely to form such relationships.

The causes of inappropriate low self-esteem are many and varied and are the root of most neurotic and psychotic signs and symptoms. Although they are in part created to enhance self-esteem, they almost invariably end up by lowering it. Fear and anxiety through their associated feelings of helplessness, guilt with its intrinsic component of worthlessness, and depression with its hopeless and helpless elements are only a few of the psychological mechanisms that can feed into feelings of inferiority.

In addition to all of these reactions, the child with minimal brain dysfunction may show any other neurotic or psychotic symptom(s) known to the child without neurological impairment. Because of his general psychological fragility, he is probably more prone to develop such psychological symptoms than the child without organic impairment. For example, instead of expressing repressed anger, he may utilize a variety of mechanisms: compulsions, phobias, nightmares, displacement, projection, and depression, just as children who are free of organic dysfunction do.

ADAPTIVE REACTIONS OF THE ADOLESCENT

Before puberty, the child with brain dysfunction may engender warm reactions in adults because he often exhibits the same appealing qualities as the normal child. Such adult responses may compensate somewhat for the rejections he sometimes suffers. In adolescence, however, these endearing qualities are lost, and he may find himself feeling more alienated than ever.

Generally during puberty,.the hyperactivity and impulsivity diminish, and he may no longer require medication for these symptoms. He becomes quieter and less aggressive. At this time he may become even more aware of how different he is from his peers. In

61

the period of life when differences from others are particularly difficult for even the normal child to handle, the child with brain dysfunction finds his dissimilarity particularly painful. He may become withdrawn and chronically depressed. His feelings of inferiority may deepen further as he dwells on his inadequacies. Other adolescents with brain dysfunction, however, do not give up the fight for acceptance. They doggedly seek friendships, ignore the subtle signs of rejection, and repress the feelings of humiliation they often suffer. Of course, these youngsters have their periods of dejection as well, when their mortifications become too overwhelming to be repressed from conscious awareness.

Like the child with brain dysfunction, the adolescent may develop a gamut of symptoms—both neurotic and psychotic—to adapt to the aforementioned basic problems. These symptoms, like all symptoms, are attempts to enhance self-esteem, diminish anxiety, and assuage the psychic pain he suffers as the result of his condition. They are, however, misguided attempts—and so they only intensify the basic problems they were designed to alleviate. He may continue to utilize some of the adaptive reactions he developed as a child. Here I describe those that typically manifest themselves in adolescence in response to the special problems youngsters with brain dysfunction are confronted with during this period of their lives.

PROBLEMS IN RELATING TO PARENTS. *Independence* vs. *Dependence*. A central problem for all adolescents is that of independence *vs.* dependence on their parents. For the adolescent with brain dysfunction this problem is particularly crucial. The normal adolescent has, or will soon have, the ability to achieve the independence he craves; the adolescent with brain dysfunction does not, and it may be a long time in coming. The normal adolescent generally achieves a certain degree of independence (not always true independence, however) through being rebellious. The adolescent with brain dysfunction cannot risk rebellion, for it implies

62

separation from his parents. He is far too dependent on them to think seriously of severing the relationship. Typically, then, he is more passive and dependent in his relationship with his parents. He compensates for the rejections he suffers in his relationships with peers by relying more heavily on his parents for affection and support. This may extend to his relationships with adults in general, with whom he often plays the role of the passive, eager-to-please child. He may thereby enjoy more gratification from adults than he does with his peers.

Parents usually recognize their responsibility to the youngster with brain dysfunction to help him develop the skills and behavioral patterns necessary to function successfully in the adult world. Generally, only a parent will have sufficient love and devotion to be willing to expend the time and energy required to achieve this goal for such children. Parents are more motivated than others to involve themselves—both intensively and extensively—in the painstaking and draining process of helping these youngsters become independently functioning adults. Although teachers, counselors, and others may provide the child with some of these growth-producing aids, their experiences with any one child are often temporary, and their involvement far less than that of a parent.

The normal adolescent relies on many individuals for a variety of gratifications. There is no single person who is vital to his existence. Even if he lost both his parents, he most often has the capacity to function effectively. This is not the case with the adolescent with brain dysfunction. His parents (especially his mother) are indispensable and irreplaceable. He cannot function without them, and generally there is no one who will assume the burden of his care with his parents' degree of patience and devotion.

Imparting the Basic Skills. The dependence *vs.* independence conflict presents a dilemma for the parents of a youngster with brain dysfunction. The more they devote themselves to helping their child, the more they may entrench his dependency. The

63

best such parents can do is to find some middle course. They should teach their child the basic skills of life and impart to him, in a step-by-step and methodical fashion, knowledge of the details of everyday living that others learn easily and often, almost unconsciously. The adolescent must be taught how to use money correctly, buy his own clothing, maintain his own bank account and checkbook, travel by bus and train, and, if possible, drive a car. He must be taught about social amenities and the subtleties of human interaction. It must not be taken for granted that he, like others, will learn these automatically in the course of his everyday living. At the same time, the goal of *independent functioning* must never be lost sight of as these skills are being taught. Not only must the parents communicate to the youngster that he is being taught these things so that he will ultimately be able to function on his own, but they must also structure situations so that he is encouraged, and often required, to *perform* self-reliantly: "If you want to buy a baseball glove with the money you've earned, you'll have to take the bus downtown and buy it yourself. We know you can do it."

The danger for parents is to allow themselves to be seduced or coerced into the overprotective role, out of sympathy for the child's pain and frustrations when he is learning to function independently. Such an attitude fosters separation anxieties in the youngster and impedes his pursuit of a life course of self-reliance.

The adolescent with brain dysfunction seeks constant reassurance from his parents. It is important that they provide him with praise for good performance; but, as already mentioned, they should direct their attention to the products of his endeavours ("Good game. Well played.") rather than provide him with generalized, often insincere, approbation ("You're a great kid."). Although most of these youngsters are exquisitely sensitive to criticism, you do them no favor by complimenting that which is obviously not praiseworthy. Similarly, when praise inevitably comes, regardless of its appropriateness, it loses its value—which is to encourage repetition of the desirable behavior. Worse, such indiscriminate approval impedes the youngster in learning to discriminate between what will be approved by those outside his home and what will not be. He then becomes even less equipped to relate adequately to others.

PROBLEMS IN RELATING TO PEERS. *The "Outsider" and the "Loner."* The adolescent with brain dysfunction often suffers his greatest mortifications in his relationships with peers. Generally, he has not learned the basic social skills that are necessary to relate successfully to normal teen-agers. He never seems to be able to say the right thing at the right time and may be ridiculed mercilessly for his ineptitude. Or more compassionate peers may look upon him as different or as someone to be pitied. Even with the latter group he is usually only tolerated or ignored—he is rarely sought out. He becomes a source of irritation to others and a source of embarrassment to his siblings (especially if they are also adolescents). Everyone seems to want to avoid him. Everyone would seem happier if he would silently disappear from the scene. Some of these adolescents withdraw in compliance with the requests that they do so, attempting to avoid the humiliations they inevitably suffer when they try to involve themselves. Others keep pushing for acceptance and desensitize themselves to their rejections. Some do not seem to be aware at all of their impact on others. It is often difficult to say whether this is the result of some intellectual defect or psychological defense mechanisms. In many, both factors are probably present.

While you naturally want your adolescent to form friendships, you must decide first whether you are going to encourage relationships with normal youngsters or with peers with brain dysfunction. Pressuring an adolescent with significant brain dysfunction to relate to normal peers may only increase his feelings of alienation and self-loathing. Only those who are close enough to the norm, who can really be expected to "fit in," should be encouraged to attempt involvements with normal adolescents.

Others should be directed to form relationships with youngsters similar to themselves. Such teen-agers are most easily found at organizations specifically established for the benefit of children with brain dysfunction. Clubs providing recreational, social, and athletic activities are often an integral part of such organizations. The specialized school or vocational training program, which the adolescent with brain dysfunction may be attending, is another possible source of appropriate companions. Lastly, you yourself can independently arrange get-togethers and social gatherings.

You can be helpful in other ways as well. One of the reasons why the adolescent with brain dysfunction has difficulty with his peers is that his repertoire of experiences is often so limited that he has little to bring into a conversation that may be of interest to others. Providing your youngster with such experiences—social, recreational, educational, etc.—enhances his likelihood of meaningful involvement with others. Dancing lessons, instruction in various sports, music lessons (especially with an instrument necessary in a rock group), and driving lessons (if he is capable) can all be helpful. Being able to drive a car may be a mixed blessing for these adolescents. It may give them a popularity they may not have otherwise enjoyed, but there is also the danger that they will be used as chauffeurs by teen-agers who have no other interest in them. Such exploitation can be terribly undermining, and the parent of such a youngster should strongly discourage it and even interdict if it is taking place. Television may provide such teen-agers with knowledge useful in social interchange. However, they easily become addicted to it, and it may then serve as a vehicle for withdrawal. Again, parental limitation is warranted.

As parents, you can be particularly helpful in the dating situation. You can play-act telephone conversations with a prospective date and provide your youngster with the various common responses and their meaning. You can teach the details of social protocol—ordering from a menu, tipping, etc. All this must be done patiently and in a step-by-step fashion with practical experiences to make the teaching more meaningful.

For many, group therapy with other adolescents with brain dysfunction can be useful. Messages from the parents can be reinforced by the group leader as well as by peers (whose opinion the adolescent usually respects and is exquisitely sensitive to). In addition, deeper and more extensive psychological problems going beyond the everyday issues dealt with here can often be helped.

Sexual Behavior and Sexual Problems. A common concern among parents is the sexual behavior of their teenager with brain dysfunction. Interestingly, the apprehension is more often about the future than the present. Typically, the parents express some surprise and relief that their adolescent with brain dysfunction isn't obsessed with sex like others his age, but fear what may happen when it does appear. Although I know of no extensive and well-documented studies on the subject, most professionals who work with these children agree that their sexual interests are more like those of a child than an adolescent. They giggle and show embarrassment over sexual matters and may exhibit some curiosity, but strong interest in sexual behavior is late in arriving and even then it seems to be of lower intensity than in the normal adolescent.

I do not believe that physiological factors play a primary role in this lag in sexual expression. Generally, the child with minimal brain dysfunction reaches puberty at about the same time as his normal peers. His growth spurt usually occurs at the normal age, as does the appearance of secondary sexual characteristics: voice changes, appearance of beard and axillary hair, etc. The same hormones responsible for these changes contribute to sexual urges. Because his physical changes are normal, I believe that psychological factors are operative in repressing the sexual urges. My guess is that, because the adolescent with brain dysfunction is less involved with his normal peers, he has fewer exposures to the stimuli that "charge up" the normal teenager. Although he is exposed as much as the normal teenager to titillating public media, he has less involvement with the more provocative and sexually exciting direct contact with peers. His fear of rejection, his anticipation of humiliation, and his awareness of his ineptitude are far greater than the normal adolescent's in the dating situation. By withdrawing and repressing his sexual drives, he protects himself from the psychic pain he would suffer were he to express himself sexually.

Masturbation, too, starts later and is generally not practiced as frequently as by the normal teen-ager. Even those parents of normal teen-agers who abhor masturbation will often prefer it to heterosexual activity with its possible consequences of promiscuity, pregnancy, and venereal disease. While the normal adolescent is generally (but not necessarily always) capable of avoiding the unfortunate consequences of his sexual activities, the adolescent with brain dysfunction may not be. Masturbation may be a far safer course for him, and the parent who discourages it, or induces guilt over it, may be performing a great disservice for such a youngster.

There are, of course, some adolescents with brain dysfunction who do have sexual problems. These run the gamut of sexual difficulties in the population at large, and there are no general recommendations I can make to cover them all. A common contributing cause is parental stimulation and encouragement —most often subtle and even unconscious. The mother who is constantly concerned that her daughter may become sexually exploited may, by her preoccupation and frequent interrogations, stimulate in the daughter an interest in these matters that might not have otherwise arisen. Such a mother may be vicariously gratifying her own wishes for sexual variety through her daughter, and the youngster's sexual acting out may be in actual compliance with the mother's basic unconscious wishes.

Similarly, the father who is exaggeratedly concerned about the possibility that his son may not be successful with girls may push him inordinately in order that the boy prove his masculinity.

The boy with brain dysfunction is generally a disappointment to his father anyway. In academics or sports he may not be able to provide the father with a sense of pride. Sex may then be selected as the area in which the father can finally gain the satisfaction that his son is truly a "man." The father then places pressures on his son to perform well sexually and may even ask him to report his "conquests." In such cases it is the father's rather than the son's, sense of masculine inadequacy that is being compensated for. By identifying with his son (who is psychologically the extension of himself), the father can gratify his own desires to achieve a sense of masculinity.

Dogmatically restrictive parental attitudes about sex may stimulate in any youngster an interest in sex that might not have otherwise been present. On the other hand, an unusually free attitude may make the youngster a misfit among his peers. Parental ignorance or misguidance about sex may also play a role in the adolescent's difficulties.

There are, of course, some adolescents with brain dysfunction who have sexual difficulties to which there has been no specific parental contribution. There are girls with brain dysfunction who can be easily exploited, and boys with brain dysfunction who make inappropriate sexual advances. Most often these boys are easily rebuffed and frightened off but occasionally their overtures can be anxiety-provoking. Their sexual advances most often have a playful or pleading quality. Mothers in the neighborhood warn their daughters to stay away from these boys—further enhancing the boys' feelings of alienation. Only rarely are the advances coercive or dangerous. These youngsters pose a significant problem for their parents. Greater parental surveillance, placement in controlled and structured situations, and group therapy may be helpful. In extreme cases, placement in a residential treatment center or psychiatric hospital may be necessary.

Problems with Drugs. It is worth reiterating that early experience with drugs, administered to alleviate the symptoms of brain dysfunction, does *not* appear to predispose these youngsters to "hard drugs" addiction when they become adolescents. Even those who have taken amphetamines since early childhood are not particularly prone to use them for "highs" when they reach their teens. Whether one will become addicted is determined far more by a predisposing psychological illness than exposure to or utilization of a medication. The youngster with brain dysfunction does not generally suffer with the constellation of psychological problems that predispose him to drug addiction. In addition, such youngsters are usually so craving for adult affection that they do not engage in the kind of rebellious behavior drug addiction usually entails.

Most adolescents with brain dysfunction do not become addicted to drugs. However, although I know of no conclusive studies on the subject, there is probably a group of adolescents with brain dysfunction who are more susceptible to the appeal of the drug culture than the normal adolescent. The child in this category is less appreciative of the remote consequences of his behavior and is so craving for acceptance that he will pay any price of admission into a group—even if that price is addiction. He may feel more comfortable in the company of the outcasts and dropouts from life who make up a signicant part of the drug culture. For the first time in his life he may have the refreshing feeling that he is not inferior to those around him. He doesn't have the ego strength to readily refuse the first dare to try drugs, and he cannot tolerate being called "chicken" if he refuses. Also his emotional pain may be so great that he may long for the desensitization or euphoria that drugs can offer.

The problem of drug addiction is an immense one and the factors that contribute to it are deeply imbedded within our social structure. Individual and even family therapeutic approaches are often ineffective because of the extensive social elements that also contribute to the problem. Guiding the adolescent with brain dysfunction along a course that will enable him to gain work and social satisfactions lessens the likelihood that he will resort to drugs. He will have less pain to anaesthetize himself to and less need for euphoric gratification. The closer he gets to leading a normal life, the less likely it will be that he gravitates toward those on the fringes of life. He must be helped to appreciate that it is more, not less, mature to refuse a foolish and dangerous dare and that not joining the majority can often be a sign of strength, rather than weakness. Again, greater parental supervision and placement in structured and well-led social, educational, and recreational situations can be helpful. Identifying with an admired leader of such a group can also be of value. Joining a therapeutic group comprised mainly (but not exclusively) of non-drug-using adolescents with brain dysfunction may also prove helpful.

Juvenile delinquency. Just as most adolescents with brain dysfunction do not become addicted to drugs, the great majority do not engage in significant delinquent behavior such as theft, assault, destruction of property, etc. There are, however, some who do become delinquent either by themselves or, more commonly, in a group. While I have no strongly confirmative statistics, there are studies that suggest that, low incidence notwithstanding, the adolescent with brain dysfunction is probably more prone to engage in delinquent behavior than his normal counterpart.

The adolescent with brain dysfunction who joins a group of delinquents does so for reasons similar to the youngster who uses drugs. His immediate craving for companionship is so great that he ignores the remote consequences of his behavior if its immediate result is group acceptance. He tends to gravitate toward, and feel comfortable with, the rejects in life who form the delinquent culture. His frequent passivity and naiveté make him a willing follower of the delinquent group's leader. However, his intellectual and social impairments may make him a poor and unreliable accomplice in any complicated scheme of antisocial behavior, and so he may not even "make it" with this group.

The delinquent youngster is, above all, an angry youngster

who is discharging his anger in maladaptive ways. Anything that can help him reduce his anger can lessen his delinquency. As already discussed, youngsters with brain dysfunction have much to be angry about: social rejection, academic deficit, neuromuscular dysfunction, etc. Any alleviation of these problems can reduce their frustration and anger. Anger related to more internal psychological difficulties has many different sources. (These vary from child to child, and it is beyond the scope of this discussion to go into them in detail.) This sort of anger may require psychotherapy if it is to be reduced. Sometimes the parents sanction delinquent behavior, overtly or covertly, in a manner similar to that described in the discussion of sexual problems. Such parents may get a kind of secret satisfaction from the adolescent's antisocial behavior, and this attitude may be revealed by their failing to restrict the youngster or punish him with conviction. Comments such as, "Joey, tell the man you're sorry," "Boys will be boys," or "He's got brain dysfunction. There's no getting through to him," have an underlying sanctioning of the antisocial behavior and can contribute to its repetition.

The delinquent adolescent with brain dysfunction, like his normal peer, is antisocial partly to build his ego by rebelling against adult authority. The parent who squelches the more innocent forms of rebellion may contribute to the youngster's resorting to more dramatic and severe types of antisocial behavior. "Way out" hairstyles and dress, which parents may not like but which are harmless, may be enough to gratify the rebellious needs of many youngsters. The parent who allows his teen-agers to express rebellion this way performs a valuable service for his youngster, and lessens the likelihood that he will resort to more extreme measures to irritate adult authority. The parent who takes away his youngster's opportunity to express himself in these innocuous ways may be unwittingly encouraging his resorting to more extreme and violent measures. I recall one fourteen-year-old whose father physically held him while the barber cut off the boy's long hair. Although previously the boy had shown poor interest in school, he became a severe truant after the hair-cutting incident.

There are other factors, as well, that may contribute to the delinquency of the adolescent with brain dysfunction. He may steal to acquire possessions to help him compensate for his feelings of deprivation (intellectual, social, etc.). Or he may use what he has stolen to bribe peers to involve themselves with him. Through ineptitude or unconscious desire he may get caught, and the resulting attention he receives may motivate him to perform other antisocial acts. It is as if he reasoned, "It is better to be punished than totally ignored." Also, his antisocial escapades may provide him with novelty and excitement in what would otherwise be a lonely, boring, and uneventful existence.

Like the drug problem, juvenile delinquency cannot be approached merely on an individual level—so extensive are the social factors that contribute to it. The same measures that are helpful for the adolescent with a drug problem may prove useful for the youngster who is delinquent: encouragement in social and recreational situations that provide healthy leadership; group therapy; and guidance into vocational and educational programs in which the adolescent with brain dysfunction is likely to be successful.

THE FUTURE. *Jobs*. The school situation, by its very nature, focuses on the major handicaps of the child with brain dysfunction. There he must learn to read, write, and master basic mathematics— things that he may be most ill-equipped to do. Work situations do not pressure him in areas in which he cannot perform well. There he has the opportunity to select the kind of job he is most suited for; the kind in which he need not fear failure; the kind that will not expose him to humiliation. For the first time in his life he may have the opportunity to succeed.

73

Aptitude testing can be helpful in determining the kind of training that will capitalize most on these youngsters' skills. There are a variety of training programs that such adolescents can enter. Sometimes they do well with a work-oriented high school curriculum where the emphasis is on vocational experiences rather than the academic. Others may do well in a standard vocational high school. Many require the more specialized vocational rehabilitation workshop or the sheltered workshop. The jobs and skills that these youngsters can be trained to do are many, and they cover the gamut of skills: electrician, repairman, bus driver, auto mechanic, plumber, construction worker, handy man, carpenter, etc. Even those whose general intelligence is borderline can be trained to function adequately in simpler vocations such as messenger, gas station attendant, guard, packer, stock clerk, etc.

The parental attitude toward the youngster's position is important in determining the commitment that he himself will have to his job. If they can appreciate that the work is intrinsically worthwhile, the chances are that their youngster will think so too. If they consider it demeaning and feel continually frustrated that he has not lived up to their anticipations, the adolescent will generally reflect their dissatisfaction in his own attitude toward his work.

With psychological support from his parents, the adolescent with brain dysfunction may find his job among the most rewarding experiences of his life. Generally, he is a willing worker, eager to follow instructions, and meticulous about attendance. He tends to be passive in his attitude toward his superiors and enjoys being considered a "good boy" by them. He is rarely among the trouble-makers or those who are agitating for change and therefore is well-liked by his bosses. He usually is fearful of asserting himself and may therefore be exploited at times. With his fellow workers, he relates better to adults (who look upon him as a "good kid") than to his peers (who may consider him a "loner" or an "oddball"). He tends to be frugal with his money and, if his parents are supporting him, may save every penny. If his social contacts are few, there will be little on which he wants to spend his earnings. Generally, he does not push for advancement and considers the job an end in itself. Supporting themselves is a reasonable goal for practically all adolescents with brain dysfunction who are of at least borderline intelligence.

There are others, however, who do not adjust as well. Their impulsivity and psychological fragility may make them ill-tempered and prone to "fly off the handle." Their judgment may be so poor that they cannot be trusted in many job situations. They appear to be so blind to the nuances of interpersonal relations that they alienate and irritate their superiors and coworkers. Such youngsters and adults do better working in sheltered work-shops under the guidance of professional personnel who are more tolerant of these anti-social manifestations than those who surround them in normal work situations.

Marriage. The self-supporting young man with minimal brain dysfunction should be able to marry. He is far better off marrying someone who has limited expectations about her husband's earning potential. Often a young lady with brain dysfunction herself makes the most suitable mate. Parental guidance and cooperation on the part of both sets of parents is most important. On occasion, the parents may have to provide steady incomes to insure financial stability for the young couple.

The young woman with brain dysfunction, if she is of at least borderline intelligence, can usually master the skills of home-making so that she can successfully manage a household. Training in these areas is best begun in adolescence, if not before. The question of her raising children is a vital one. Many are quite capable of doing so. Those who are not may not be able to adequately use contraceptive devices either. In cases where it is obvious that a young adult may never be able to adequately care for a child, probably the most humane course is sterilization.

Since our recognition of this disorder is so recent, few professionals have had much experience with the marital situation of those who have brain dysfunction. As more of these youngsters marry, our knowledge will increase and we will be in a better position to advise those in this category.

In closing, I would like to emphasize that no one can predict with certainty how any given child will grow up. The aforementioned difficulties are some of the more common; but there are many children with minimal brain dysfunction who do not have any of them. There are many adolescents whom I have seen in my practice whose psychological tests and clinical reports from earlier years were replete with pathological manifestations; and yet as adolescents they presented with so few difficulties that I found it hard to believe that I was reading about the same youngster, and there are others, whom I myself have observed over the years, who have improved so significantly that by the time they reached adolescence no one would consider them to be different from other youngsters their age. The parent, therefore, who sees the label of minimal brain dysfunction as condemning a child to irreparable and lifelong psychological disorder, not only may carry an unnecessary burden himself but may contribute to the child's pessimistic outlook as well—thereby impeding the progress he might otherwise have made.

Part Two
For Boys and Girls

Introduction for Boys and Girls

My name is Dr. Richard Gardner. I am a child psychiatrist. For those of you who don't know what that is, a child psychiatrist is a special kind of doctor who tries to help children who have troubles and worries.

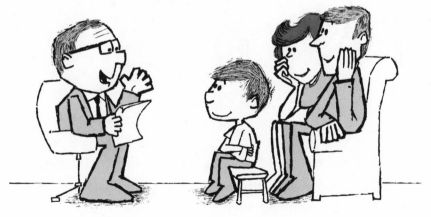

Some of the children who are brought to see me have what is called *minimal brain dysfunction*.

In this book I am going to tell you many things about minimal brain dysfunction. Children with this trouble have taught me a lot about what they think and feel and what they can do to help themselves.

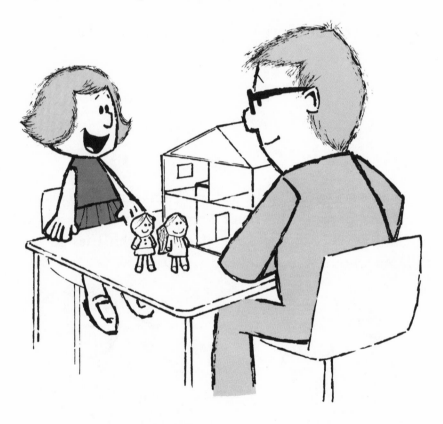

I have written this book so that other children with brain dysfunction can be helped by the things these children and I have learned together.

WHEN SOMETHING SAD OR PAINFUL HAPPENS TO YOU

I'd like to tell you a few things before we start talking about brain dysfunction. When something happens that's sad and painful, usually the best thing for you to do is to try to find out exactly what the trouble is. Then it is easier for you to decide what to do to help yourself feel better. Some children don't do this. Instead, they make believe that nothing's wrong, or they try to hide their sadness. When they do this, they are not trying to help themselves, and so their problems usually are not solved, and . . .

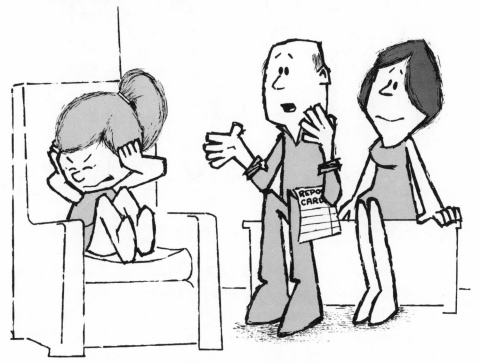

. . . they may even get worse. It's much better to know the truth about your problems than to hide from them, even though the truth can often be frightening or painful. When you know the truth, you can often do something about your troubles. If you hide from the truth, you can do nothing about your problems, and so things usually get worse.

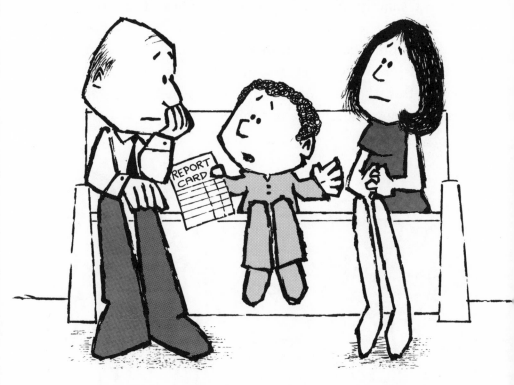

Some boys and girls do this with the troubles they have about their brain dysfunction. If such children stopped hiding from their problems and started trying to do something about them, they'd most often feel better about things. If you've been doing this, now's the time to stop!

HOW TO USE THIS BOOK

In this book I try to help children understand more about brain dysfunction and to give them advice about some of the things they can do to help themselves. I'll talk about many of the usual problems that boys and girls with brain dysfunction have. Some of the problems will be like the ones you have, others will not. I'll talk about many problems. Don't try to read too much at once. Read each part carefully and make sure you understand everything that's said. Many children like to read this book along with their mother or father.

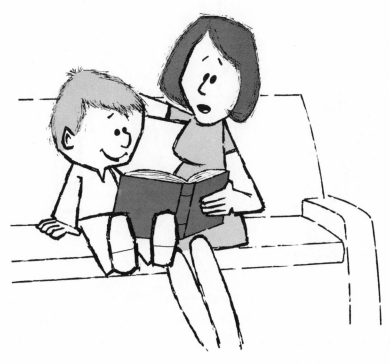

I think that's a very good idea because then your mother or father is right there to answer any questions you may have. If you don't understand something, it's very important to ask your parent to explain it to you. Don't be ashamed to ask the same question over and over again—until you understand it. Most mothers and fathers are very happy to explain things to you in order to make them clear.

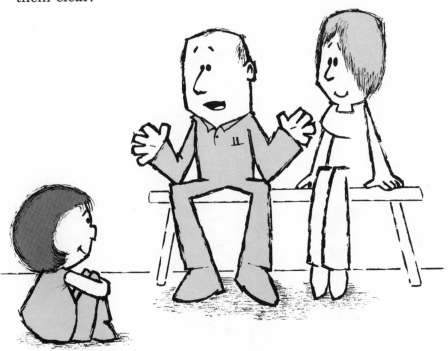

If you read this book carefully—think about the things I have said—talk to your parents about them—and try to do the things I have suggested—I think you'll feel better about your problems.

What the Brain Does

First, I am going to tell you a few things about the brain.

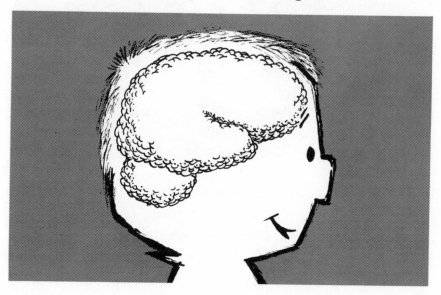

As you know, the brain is a part of the body that is inside the head.

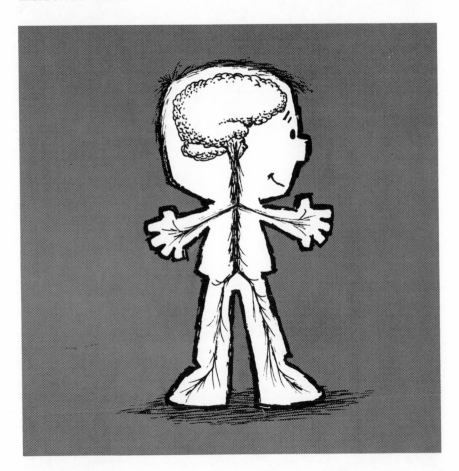

The brain is connected to almost every part of the body by the nerves. Nerves, like wires, connect the brain to the different parts. By sending electric signals through a nerve, the brain controls the movement of the part of the body that the nerve is connected to.

The brain can do many interesting and wonderful things.

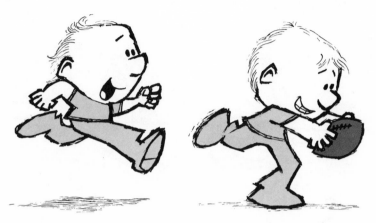

When you run and play ball, it is your brain that controls the movement of your arms and legs. It does this by sending signals through the nerves that go from the brain to the arms and legs. Most often, it does this in such a way that you don't even have to think about it.

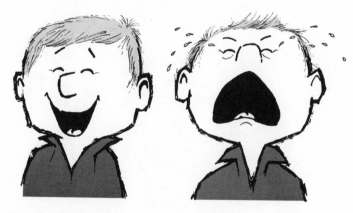

In the same way, when you laugh or cry . . .

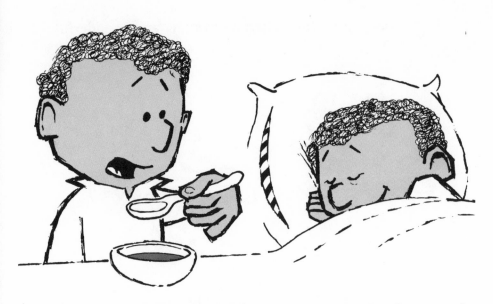

. . . eat or sleep, it is your brain that controls what you do.

When you read, it is your brain that helps you understand what the words mean.

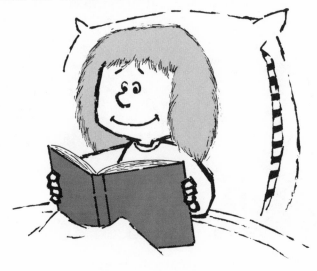

It also helps you figure out arithmetic problems.

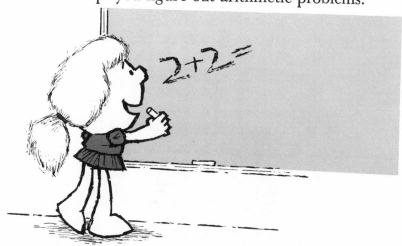

When you write, it is your brain that gets your fingers to write the letters in the correct way. It does this by sending electric signals through the nerves that go from the brain to the hand and fingers.

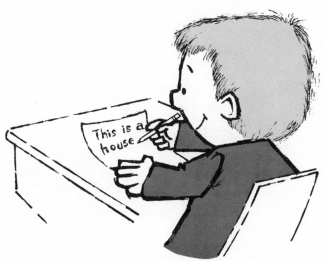

When you talk . . .

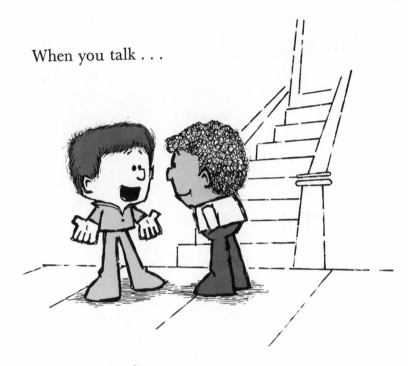

. . . and when you sing . . .

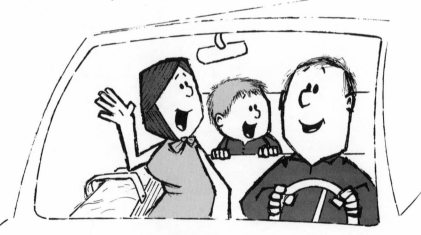

. . . your brain helps you get the words out right.

90

The brain helps you understand what you see . . .

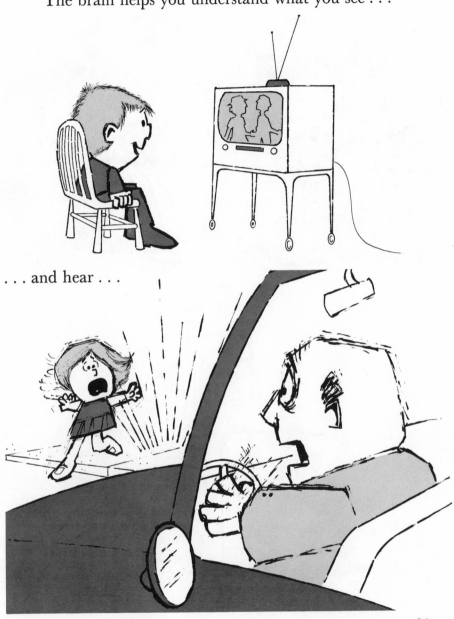

. . . and hear . . .

. . . and feel . . .

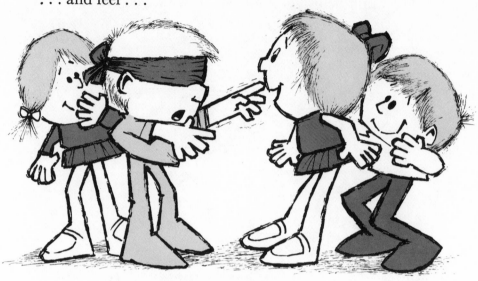

. . . and taste . . .

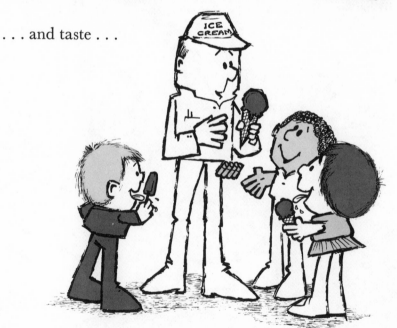

92

. . . and smell.

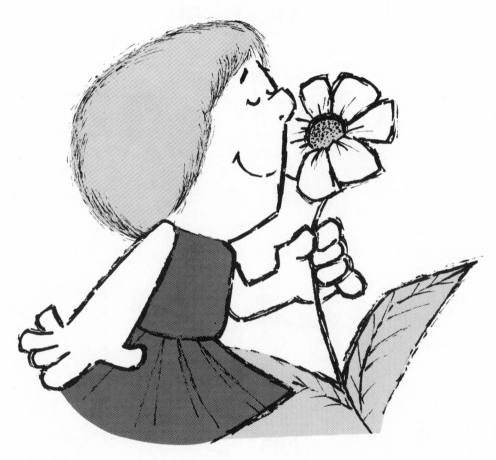

It also helps you remember things like songs . . .

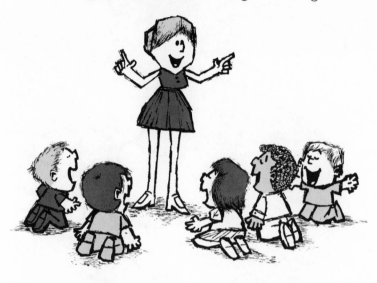

. . . and how to dress yourself.

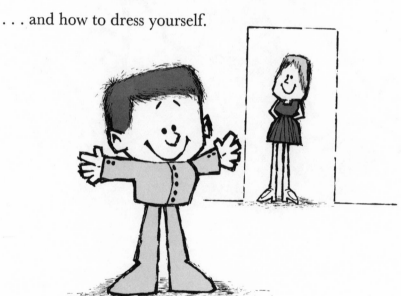

Your brain helps you understand jokes . . .

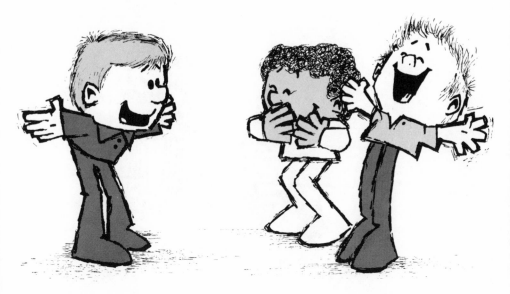

. . . and games.

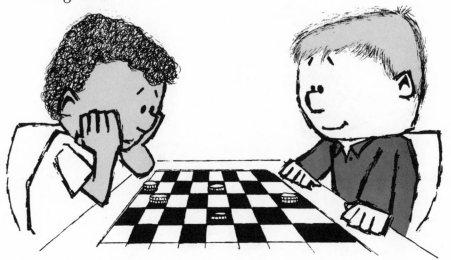

It makes you feel good when things go right . . .

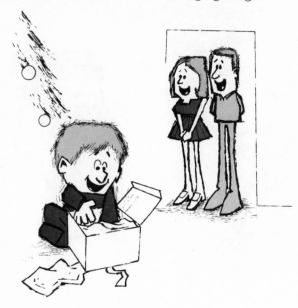

. . . and bad when things go wrong.

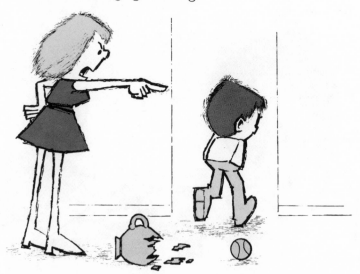

There are many other interesting and wonderful things the brain can do. I think I have told you enough to give you a good idea about some of them.

One important thing to remember about the brain is that it does many different kinds of things.

People Are Different in Many Ways

As you know, not everybody is the same.

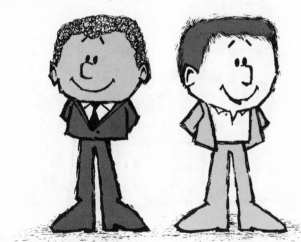

Some people have dark skin and some have light skin.

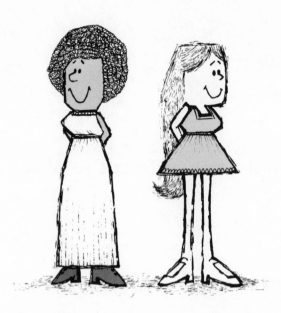

Some have curly hair and some have straight hair.

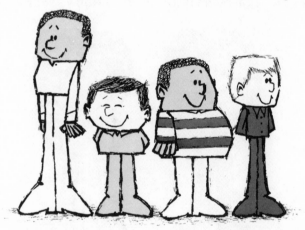

Some are tall and some are short; some are fat and some are thin.

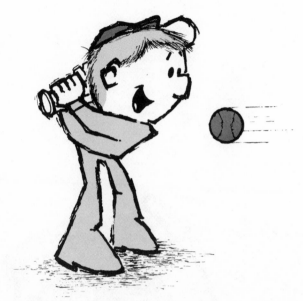

Certain people are good at baseball but cannot swim.

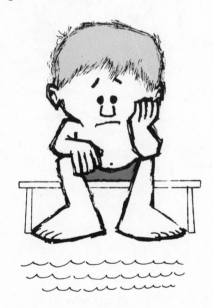

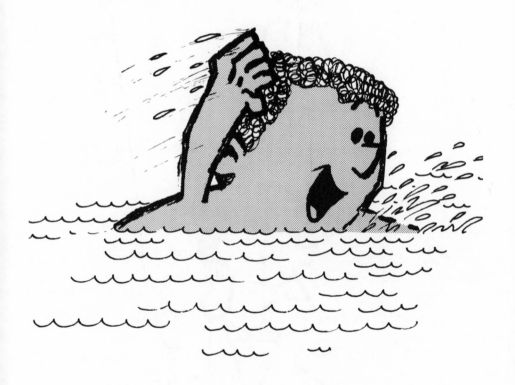

Others may be good at swimming . . .

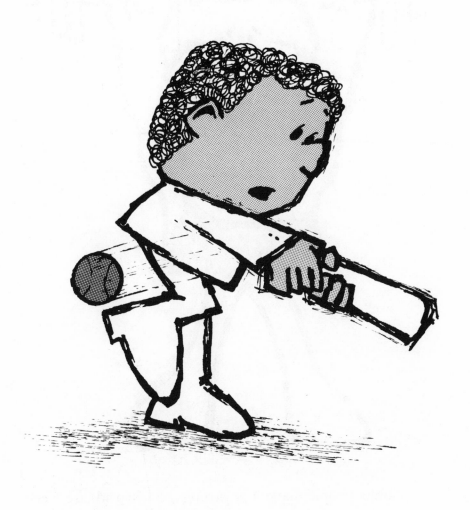

. . . but cannot play baseball too well.

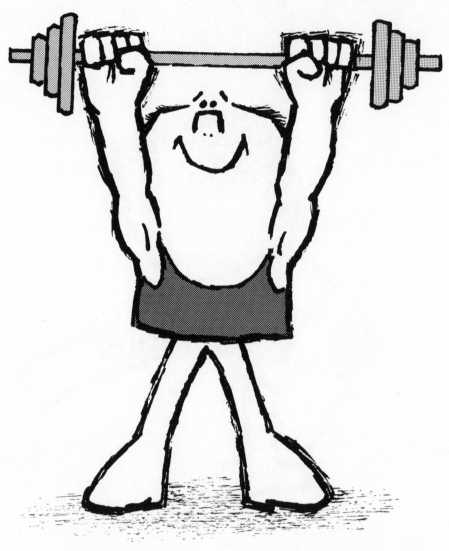

Some people have big strong hands and are very good at picking up heavy things, but cannot use their hands to play the piano or make a fine watch. Others have small hands; and although they are not very strong, they might be very good at sewing or making model airplanes.

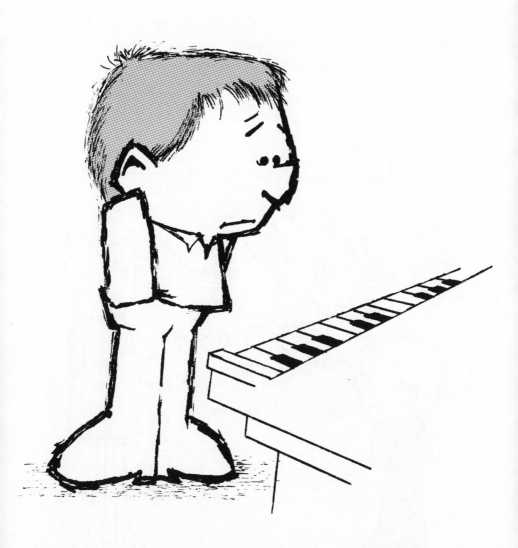

So you see, people are all different. Most people are good in some things and poor in others. Nobody is good in everything, but practically everybody has some things that he can do well.

As with other parts of the body, people's brains are different, too. Some have brains with very good memories, and some have poor memories.

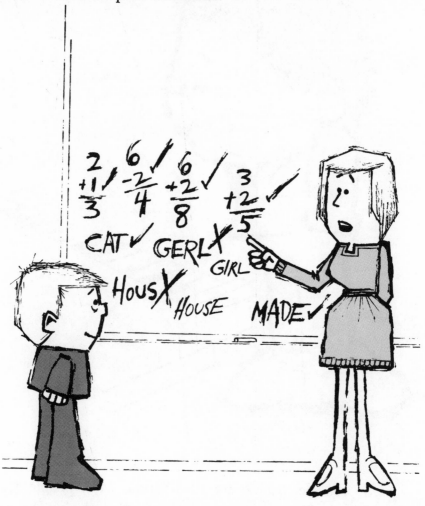

Some people are good at arithmetic, but very poor in spelling.

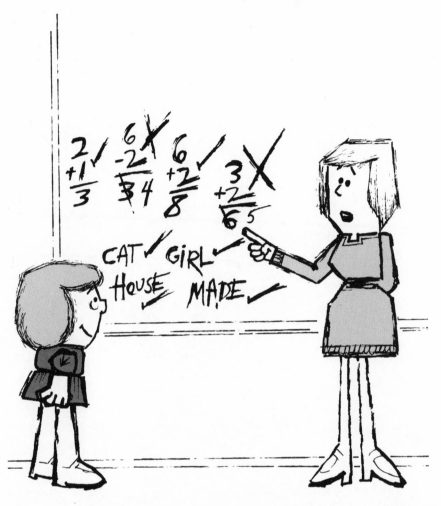

Others are poor in arithmetic, but good in spelling.

I hope now that you have a good idea about the kinds of things the brain can do and how different people have different kinds of brains.

What Is Brain Dysfunction?

Now I would like to tell you about minimal brain dysfunction.

In some children one or a few small parts of the brain do not work well. Another way to say this is that their brains do not function well. *Work well* and *function well* mean the same thing. *Dysfunction* means *not* working well or *not* functioning well. *Not working well* and *dysfunction* mean the same thing. A child with brain dysfunction is a child whose brain is not working well.

Minimal means just a little bit. When a child has minimal brain dysfunction a little bit of his brain is not working well. The rest of his brain is working fine. Since only a small part of the brain isn't working well, such a child has trouble with one or a few of the many things that the brain does.

109

HOW CHILDREN GET MINIMAL BRAIN DYSFUNCTION

Now you may be wondering how children get minimal brain dysfunction. First, some are just born that way. There may be people in their families—a mother, a father, an uncle, or an aunt—who were born that way too. For example, this boy has trouble with his handwriting.

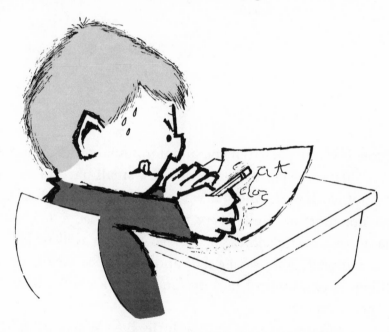

He had an uncle who also had a very poor handwriting as a boy, but the uncle's handwriting got better as he got older. However, the uncle had to work extra hard to make his handwriting better. This boy will have to work extra hard too if he is to improve his handwriting.

Some children get brain dysfunction from a sickness their mother had while they were still inside her—before they were born.

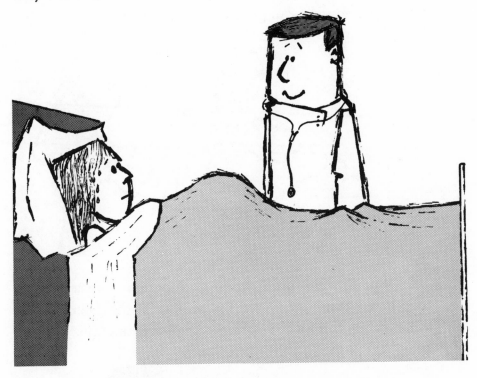

The little baby inside this lady may get the same sickness she has. If the sickness goes to the baby's brain, he may get brain dysfunction.

There are some babies who come out of their mother too early. Instead of staying inside nine months, like most babies, they may come out one, two, or even three months too early. Such babies are called "premature babies." Some, but not all, premature babies have brain dysfunction.

111

Sometimes, while an infant is being born, his head has trouble coming out of his mother's vagina. His head may be so squeezed that his brain may get hurt. This is one way that boys and girls can get brain dysfunction.

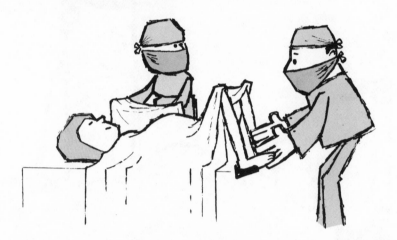

Some children get brain dysfunction from a sickness they had when they were very young. If the sickness goes to his brain, this child might get brain dysfunction.

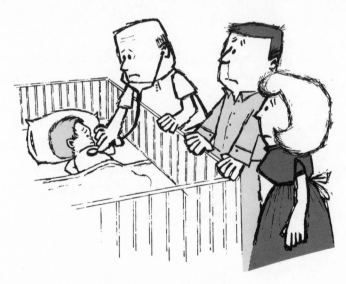

Some boys and girls get it from an illness they had when they were older. When such an illness goes to the brain, the child may have brain dysfunction.

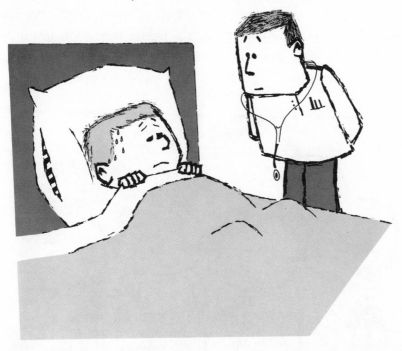

Some children get it from being struck on the head.

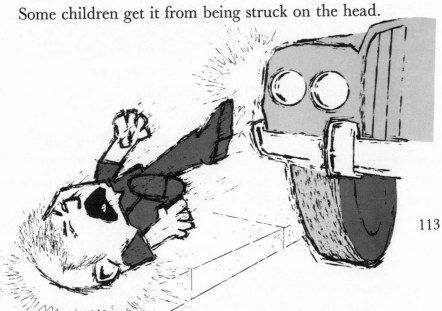

113

This is why children with brain dysfunction are sometimes called *brain injured* or *brain damaged*. But this is a poor name because very few of all the children who have brain dysfunction got that way because they were struck on the head. Of all these children with brain dysfunction, only one got that way from being struck on the head. All the others got it in one of the other ways I have just talked about.

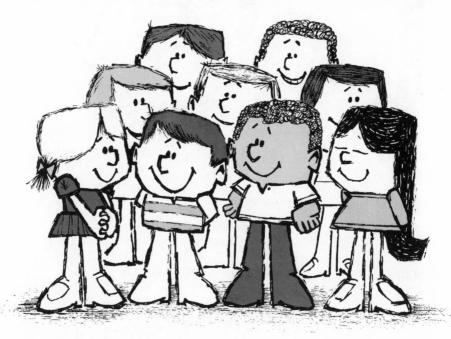

There are many children who have minimal brain dysfunction and no one—not even a doctor—knows the cause. They still have minimal brain dysfunction because a small part or a few small parts of their brain do not work well. As time goes on, doctors will learn more and more about the causes of brain dysfunction in these children.

114.

An important thing to remember is that no matter how you got brain dysfunction—whether you were born with it —or got it from an illness—or got it from being struck on the head—or even when the cause is not known—you can usually be helped. The troubles you have are most often treated in the same way, no matter what the cause. However, in order for you to learn some things, you need more help and will have to work harder than most other children.

The Kinds of Trouble Children with Brain Dysfunction Have

Now I would like to tell you about some of the troubles and problems that children with brain dysfunction sometimes have. You might have some of these troubles and problems yourself.

A very important thing to remember about these troubles is that most of them get better as time goes on. It is also important to remember that most of these problems can be helped.

SOME DO CERTAIN THINGS LATER THAN OTHERS

Some boys and girls with brain dysfunction learn to do certain things later than others their own age. For example, most children start to walk when they are between ten and fourteen months old. Children with brain dysfunction might not start to walk until later. However, even though such children might start late, most do walk. And when they do, most walk as well as any other child. Many walk so well that even a doctor might not be able to tell the difference between them and children who started to walk at the usual age.

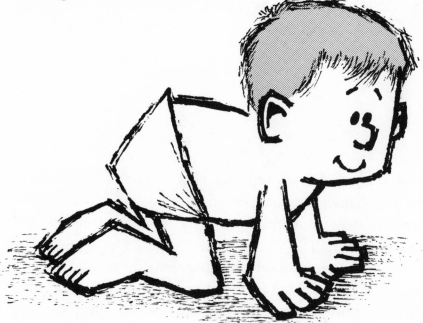

This boy with brain dysfunction could not walk when he was one year old.

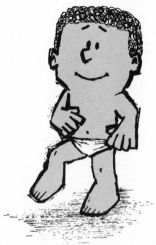

This boy does not have brain dysfunction, and he was walking a little when he was one year old.

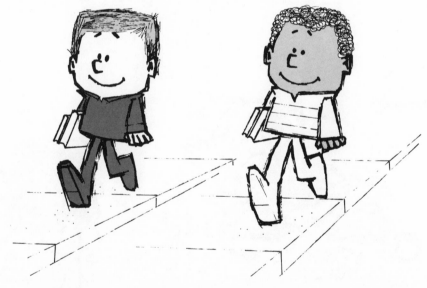

Both boys are older now, and both walk equally well. No one could tell that the boy with brain dysfunction started late.

Most children start to talk between the ages of one and two. A child with brain dysfunction might not start to talk until later. But this same child, when he gets older, might be able to speak just as well as the child who started to speak earlier.

Also, remember that the child who is later than others in doing *some things* is not later than *everyone else* in *everything*. He may even do some things earlier than others. For example, this girl with brain dysfunction didn't talk as well as others her age.

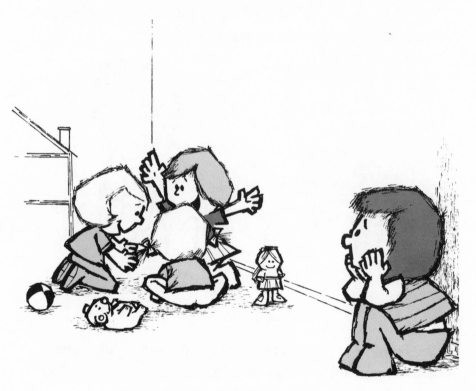

However, she could string beads far better than her friends.

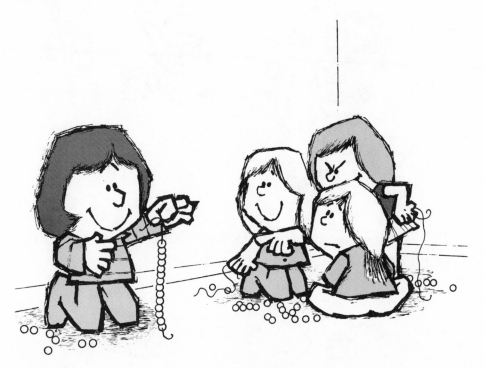

This boy was late in learning how to ride his tricycle.

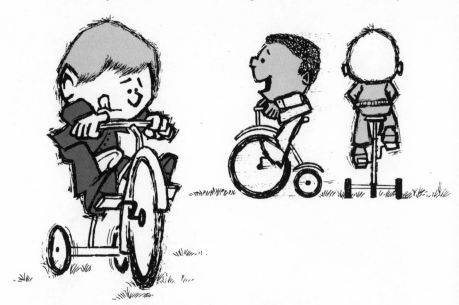

However, he could do puzzles much earlier than the same boys who rode their tricycles well.

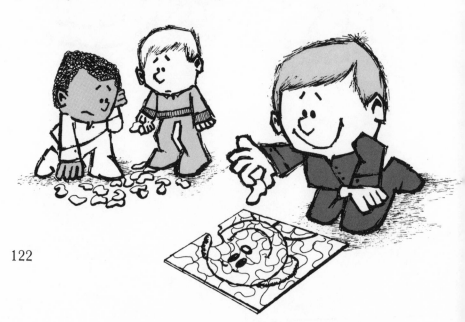

This is true of many of the troubles that children with brain dysfunction have. You may be later in starting to do certain things and take a longer time to learn them, but you will probably finally learn and catch up to the others.

SOME CAN'T DO CERTAIN THINGS AS WELL AS OTHERS

There are many different kinds of troubles that boys and girls with brain dysfunction have. This is because the brain does many things, and usually one or a few of its parts are not working well. The rest of the brain is usually working quite well.

Some children with brain dysfunction have trouble reading. Others read quite well, but have difficulty with writing or spelling.

Some can't draw too well.

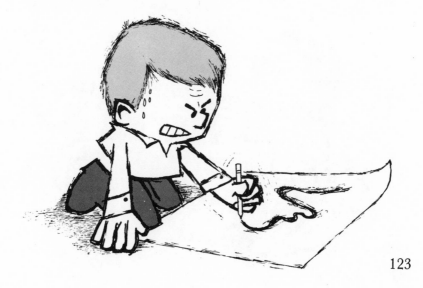

Others may draw beautifully . . .

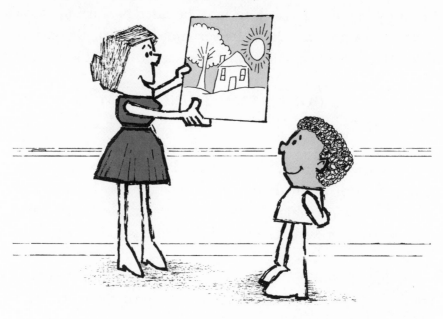

. . . but have trouble catching a ball.

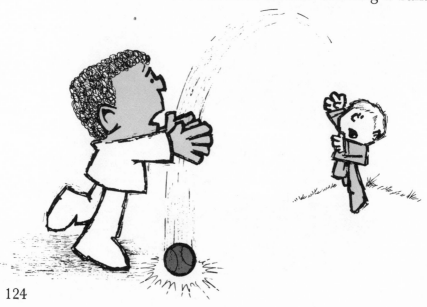

Some are very active. They run around a lot and just can't sit still very long. Many cannot pay attention to one thing for very long and find that their minds wander.

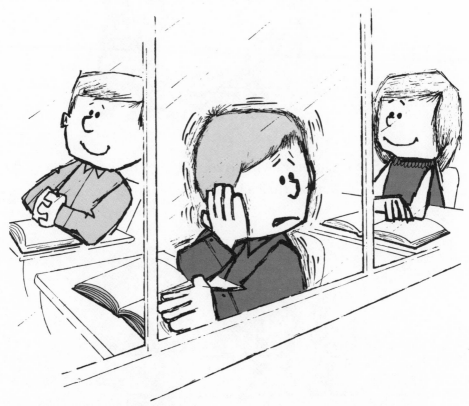

However, many boys and girls with brain dysfunction pay attention quite well.

Some have trouble understanding the rules of the games they play with other children. Others do this quite well.

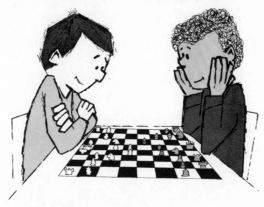

Some children with brain dysfunction can't tie their shoelaces or button their clothing, while other children their age can.

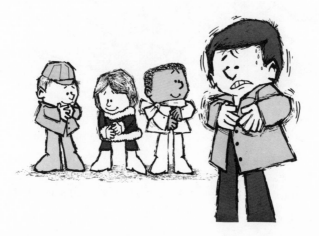

However, there are other children with minimal brain dysfunction who do these things without any difficulty.

Certain boys and girls with brain dysfunction easily get upset over the smallest things. They would like not to get so upset, but they just can't seem to help it. It is harder for them to learn to control themselves.

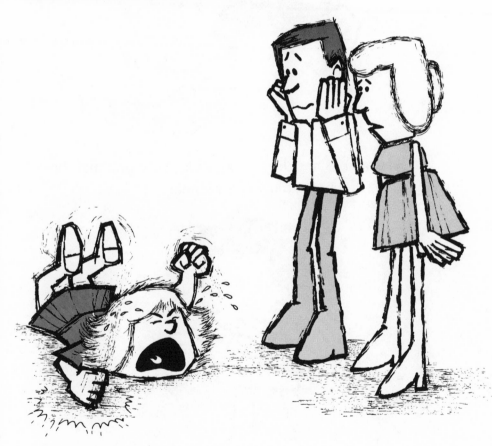

Some have poor memories and have to work very hard to make things stick in their minds.

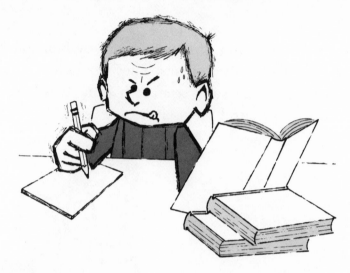

Although some boys and girls with minimal brain dysfunction do not do too well in school . . .

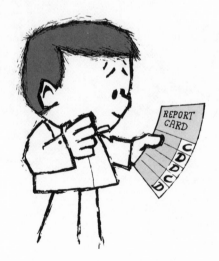

... others may be among the best students in their class.

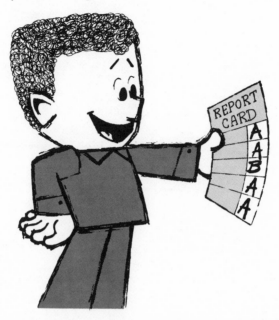

There are other troubles that children with minimal brain dysfunction may have, but I have told you about the most common ones. Most children with brain dysfunction have one or only a few of these difficulties. It is very rare to see a child with all of the problems I have just told you about.

I think that now you have a good idea about the kinds of trouble that children with brain dysfunction have.

How Children with Brain Dysfunction Can Be Helped and What They Can Do to Help Themselves

Now I would like to tell you about those things which can be done to help children who have brain dysfunction. There are many boys and girls with brain dysfunction who think that nothing can be done for them. This is just not so.

MOST CHILDREN GET BETTER AS THEY GET OLDER

First, even without the things I am going to tell you about, most children with brain dysfunction get better and better as they get older. As I have already told you, children with brain dysfunction often do things later than other

131

children. But as they grow older, they catch up to the others in many things. However, you don't want to just sit and wait. There are things you can do to help yourself catch up faster.

SPECIAL CLASSES FOR CHILDREN WITH BRAIN DYSFUNCTION

There are special classes for boys and girls with brain dysfunction. These classes are not found everywhere. But every year more and more classes are starting.

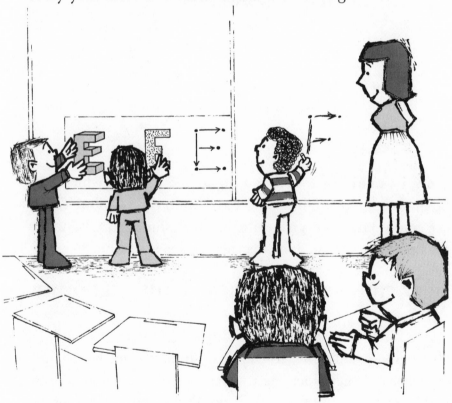

In these special classes, there are teachers who know how to help children with brain dysfunction learn the best way possible. The classes often have very few children. Then each child can be given special attention and be taught in the way that is best for him.

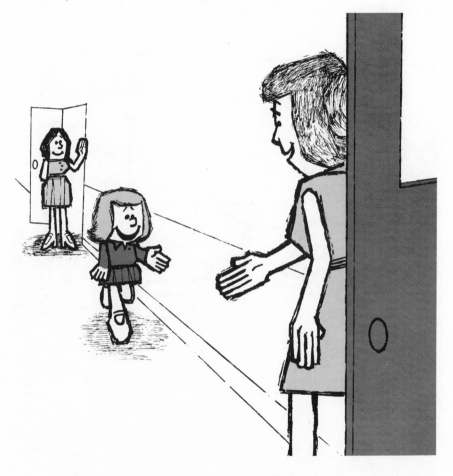

Many children start off in these special classes and then learn well enough to go on to regular classes.

SPECIAL TEACHERS FOR CHILDREN WITH BRAIN DYSFUNCTION

There are special teachers who help children with different kinds of problems. Those children who have trouble speaking can often be helped by a speech teacher.

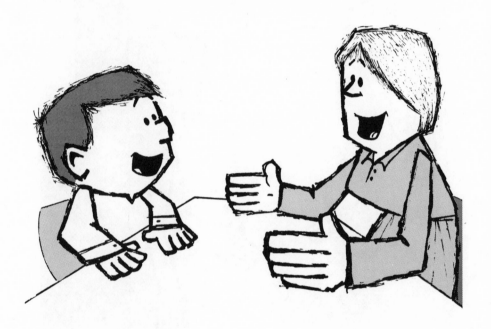

Other teachers are very good at helping boys and girls who may have trouble reading or writing.

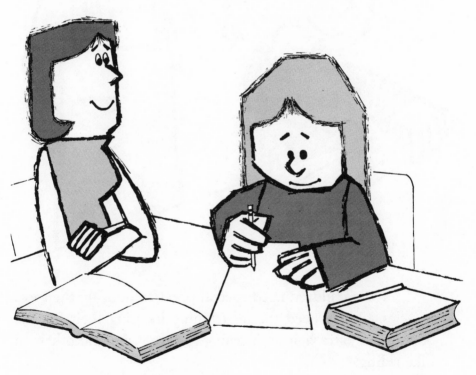

Children who have trouble using their arms and legs correctly can be helped with special games or exercises.

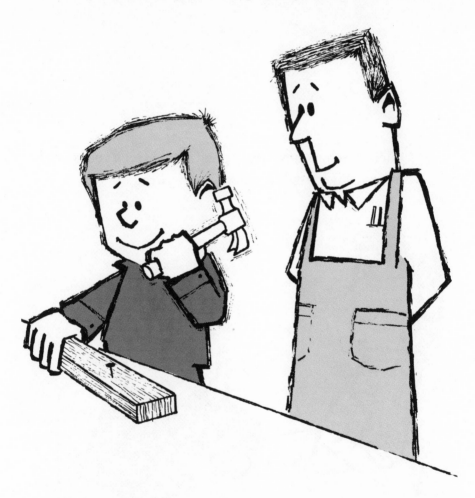

Some children need special practice in using their eye muscles. Others need special training in using their fingers. Some need extra help in learning how to swim and others in bike riding.

THINGS YOU CAN DO TO HELP YOU LEARN BETTER

Most children with brain dysfunction have some trouble learning. You may have to study harder and longer than other children. It's best for you to study in a place that is very quiet. You may find that it's very hard for you to concentrate on your homework if a TV set is on or if children are playing nearby. It's hard for *all* children to study when there's lots of noise around them, but it's even harder for children with minimal brain dysfunction.

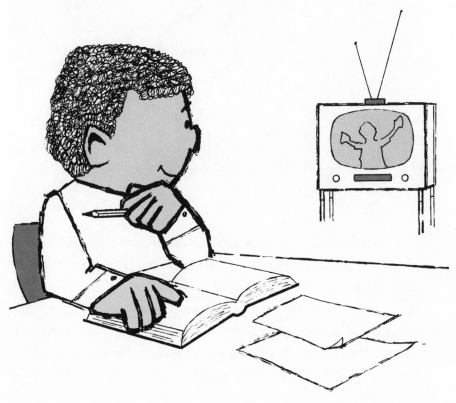

Most children with brain dysfunction, like all other children, find they study best in a quiet room at a table or desk with nothing on it except their school work. It's also easier to concentrate when the window shades are pulled down.

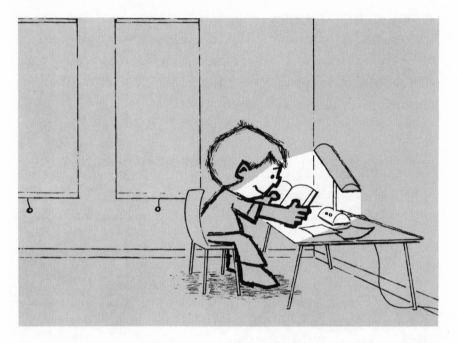

Many children with brain dysfunction, like most other children, find that they can learn best early in the morning, when they are most alert and when their minds are clear. So, on Saturday or Sunday, you might try doing a little studying right after you get up—before you go out and play. During the week, it might be a good idea to rest about fifteen minutes in a dark, quiet room before doing your homework.

MEDICINES SOMETIMES HELP

There are certain medicines that sometimes help children with brain dysfunction.

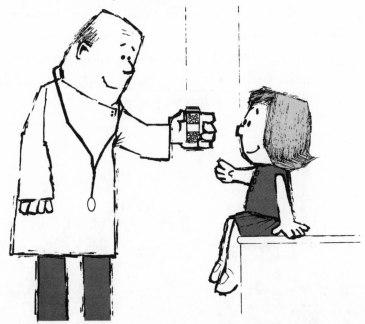

Doctors now have many pills that may be helpful. These medicines sometimes help children stay calm, remember things, and keep their minds on what they are doing. There are many different kinds of pills, and the doctor must try to find out which ones work best for each child.

Since children are different, a pill that works well for one child might not work for another. Your doctor has to try a few and see which ones work best for you. Not all children need pills, and your doctor can decide if you need them.

SPECIAL CLUBS FOR CHILDREN WITH BRAIN DYSFUNCTION

Many cities and towns have special clubs for children with brain dysfunction. It's very important to join a club like this if there is one near you. There you can meet other boys and girls with brain dysfunction and do many things with them. In such clubs they have sports, arts and crafts, games, and many other interesting activities.

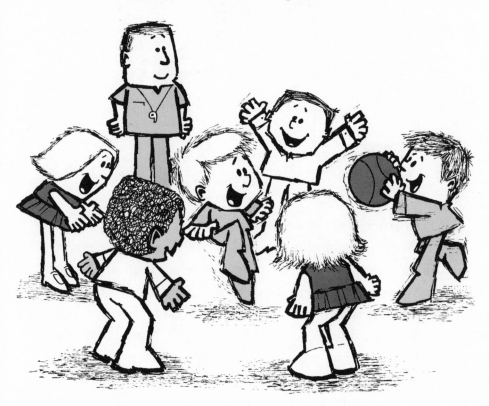

Most children with brain dysfunction feel better about themselves at such clubs because they see that they aren't the only ones with problems but that there are many others with similar difficulties. And so it helps them feel less different. Also, the children at these clubs will often be more friendly with children who have brain dysfunction because they have brain dysfunction themselves.

As you can see, there are many things that can be of help to children with brain dysfunction. However, such a child has to work harder and do many things on his own if he is to be helped in the best way possible.

Worries that Children with Brain Dysfunction Often Have

There are some boys and girls with brain dysfunction who become very upset about their difficulties. Just because one or a few small parts of their brains do not work well, they think that *everything* about themselves is no good.

Some are scared to be with other children because they can't play certain games as well, or run as fast, as some of the others.

143

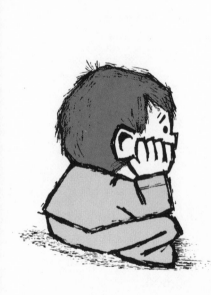

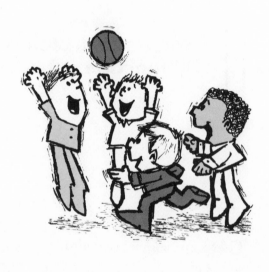

Many become very sad because they think they will always be that way. They do not know the things I have just told you: how they can be helped, how they can help themselves, and how things get better as they grow older.

SOME CHILDREN WITH BRAIN DYSFUNCTION WORRY ABOUT BEING RETARDED

Many children with brain dysfunction fear that they are retarded. Let me tell you something about what the word *retarded* means.

Of all children with brain dysfunction, there are a few who have so much trouble learning that they have been given a special name. They are called retarded children. Most children with minimal brain dysfunction are *not* retarded. A child with minimal brain dysfunction has trouble in only one or a few parts of his brain, and so he has trouble doing only a few things. The retarded child has more things the matter with his brain, and so he has more problems —especially in learning. The retarded child has so much trouble learning so many different kinds of things that he needs to be in a class different from the kind needed by the child with minimal brain dysfunction. He cannot learn as well, so he needs a different kind of class.

The retarded child learns *most* things more poorly than other children his age. The child with minimal brain dysfunction learns some things *more poorly*, some things *equally well*, and some things *even more quickly* than others his age. As I have told you, some children with brain dysfunction are among the best in their class. The retarded child has too many troubles learning to be among the best in his class.

145

Sometimes boys and girls with minimal brain dysfunction think they are retarded when they really are not. Many worry about this, and feel very sad, because they think they are retarded. Most of the children who worry this way are *not* retarded. In addition, it is important to remember that even those children who are retarded are not backward in everything.

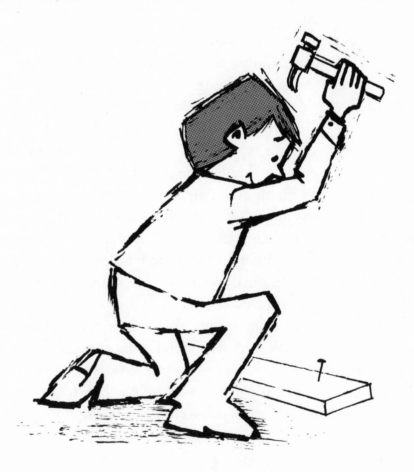

Many retarded children can learn interesting and wonderful things and . . .

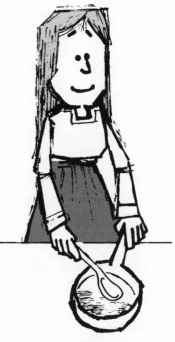

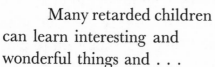

can lead useful lives when they grow up.

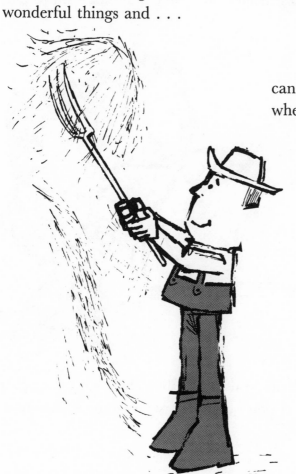

WHAT YOU CAN DO IF OTHER CHILDREN ARE CRUEL TO YOU

Most boys and girls with brain dysfunction have problems with children who do not have brain dysfunction. Most children, at times, call one another bad names. I'm sure you have done it, at times. However, children can sometimes be very cruel, and they may make fun of a child with brain dysfunction. They may think that the child with brain dysfunction is strange, and they may not want to play with him.

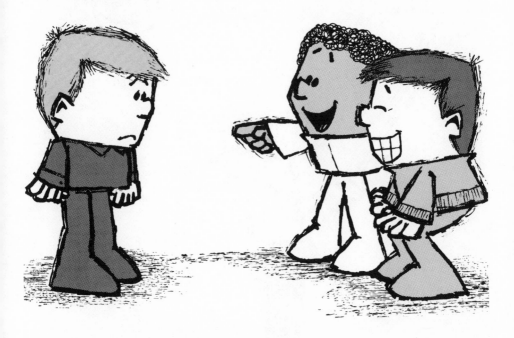

Now, what can you do if other children are cruel to you or make fun of you because of your brain dysfunction?

THERE'S SOMETHING WRONG WITH SOMEONE WHO MAKES FUN OF THE CHILD WITH BRAIN DYSFUNCTION

First, it's important to remember that there must be something wrong with someone who makes fun of a person just because he has brain dysfunction.

This girl had trouble learning in school. One day, some children laughed at her and called her stupid. She answered, "There must be something wrong with you if you can laugh at someone who has trouble learning." The children were then ashamed about what they had done and stopped calling her names.

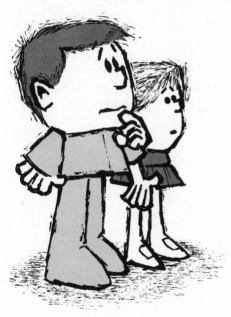 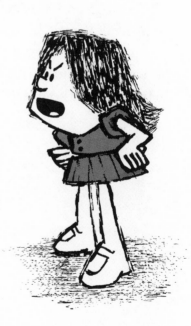

THE THINGS OTHER CHILDREN SAY ABOUT YOU MAY SOMETIMES BE TRUE

All children, even those without brain dysfunction, are sometimes teased. If children do call you names, it's important to ask yourself if it's true what they are saying. Although there is no excuse for children to call you names and although it's cruel of them to do so, what they say may still be true and you may be able to learn something about yourself that may be helpful to you.

Children were always calling this boy, "Baby." When he would go out to play, they often said to him things like, "Here comes the baby!" or "Look at the baby!"

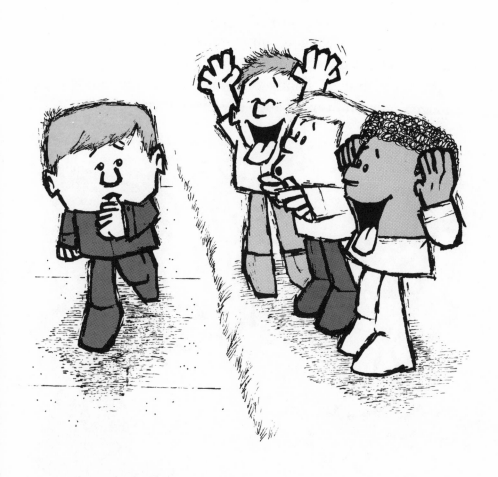

151

Although it wasn't nice of the other children to laugh at him, it was true that he often acted younger than he was. He sucked his thumb, was often very silly, spoke in a baby way, and cried very easily. After he thought about what the children were saying to him, he decided to try and stop acting like a baby. It took him a long time, and he had to try very hard, but he finally did stop. Then, the children no longer called him baby and they played with him.

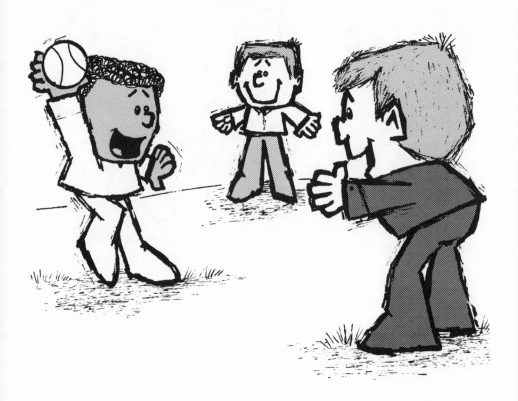

THE THINGS OTHER CHILDREN SAY ABOUT YOU MAY NOT BE TRUE

However, it's also important to remember that what other children may say about you may *not* be true.

This boy thought that every bad thing that anyone ever said about him was true. Children laughed at him sometimes because he couldn't speak too well, and they would sometimes call him stupid.

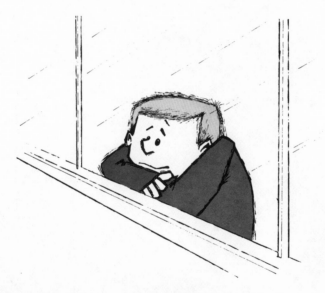

Actually, he was very smart, but his brain dysfunction caused him to have trouble speaking. Otherwise he was perfectly all right. But when the children called him stupid, he thought he must be stupid. He didn't think that it could be possible that they might be wrong. If he had realized that they were wrong, he would not have felt so sad.

153

BAD NAMES CANNOT HURT YOU

Another important thing to know is that being called names cannot really hurt you. No matter what other children *say* about you, it cannot really hurt you. There is an old saying: "Sticks and stones may break my bones . . .

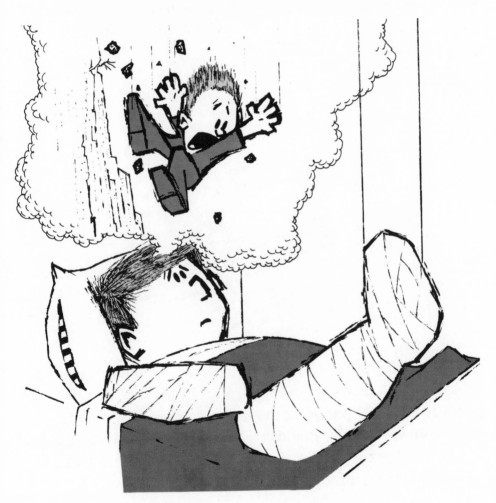

. . . but names will never hurt me."

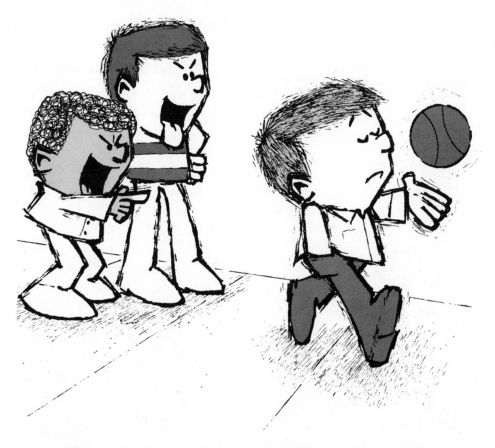

This saying is a good answer to children who make fun of you for any reason.

SOMEWHERE THERE ARE FRIENDS FOR EVERYONE

There will always be some children who will not like you no matter who you are and what you do, and no matter how hard you try to be friendly. Even children without brain dysfunction are not liked by everybody. Just because some children may not like you does not mean that no one will ever like you. There are many people who can like you even though you have only a few friends now. One place to find such friends is at the clubs for children with brain dysfunction.

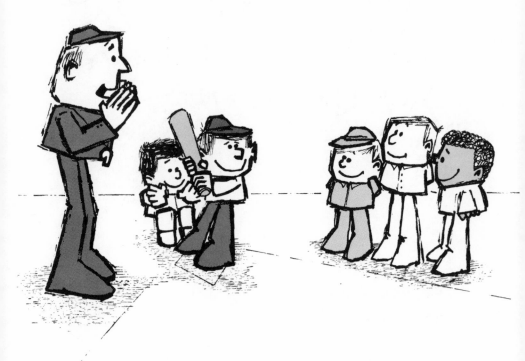

Since all the children in these clubs have brain dysfunction, they usually do not make fun of one another. The special classes for children with brain dysfunction is another good place to find friends. However, you can't just sit back and expect friends to come to you. You have to go out where other people are, be friendly, and work at making friendships.

It's important to remember that the main thing that other children care about is whether you're nice and how much fun it is to be with you. If you play well with them and are friendly, most children will want to play with you even though you have brain dysfunction. Even if they call you names once in a while, they'll like you and want to be with you if you are a friendly person.

This boy used to get very upset and cry if he made the smallest mistake when he played baseball.

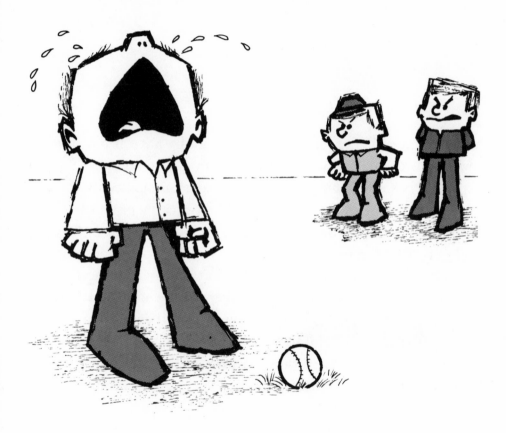

The others didn't mind his mistakes as much as they minded his crying, so they stopped asking him to play with them. They didn't mind the mistakes he made once in a while. Everybody makes mistakes once in a while. They were bothered by his crying.

When he was able to control himself from crying each time he made a mistake, the others started asking him to play again.

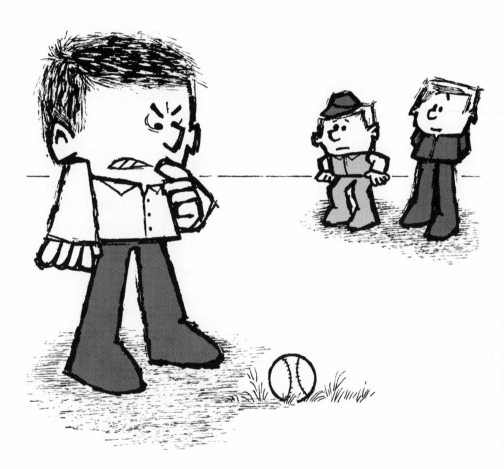

ONLY A SMALL PART OF YOU ISN'T WORKING WELL

Many boys and girls with brain dysfunction feel very bad about themselves. One reason for this is that they think that everything about themselves is no good just because one or a few small parts of their brain are not working well. Those who understand that only a small part of themselves isn't working well will feel better about themselves.

YOU CAN'T GET BRAIN DYSFUNCTION FROM BEING BAD

Some children think that they got their brain dysfunction from being bad.

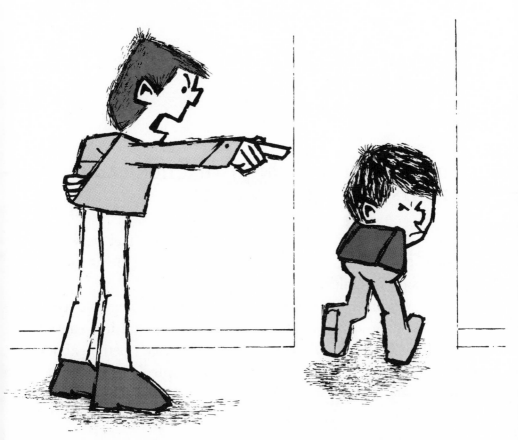

All children are bad at times, but no child ever got brain dysfunction from being bad. Before, I told you about some of the things that cause brain dysfunction. As I am sure you remember, badness was not one of them. Those children who think that they got brain dysfunction from being bad often think that if they had been very good, they would not have gotten brain dysfunction. When these children come to realize that they didn't get brain dysfunction from being bad, they often feel better about themselves.

CHILDREN WITH BRAIN DYSFUNCTION CAN'T ALWAYS CONTROL THEMSELVES

Some children with brain dysfunction feel very bad about themselves because they cannot control themselves as well as other children.

When these children learn that their trouble controlling themselves is not all their fault, but that it is caused by their brain dysfunction, they often feel better about themselves. Then, if they are able to control themselves at times—by trying very hard—they get to feel better about themselves.

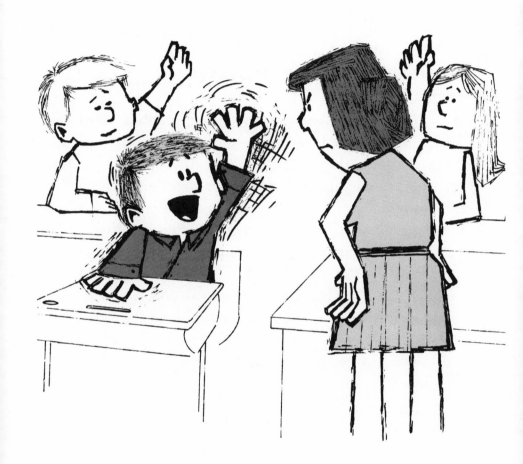

THE FEAR OF MAKING MISTAKES

The more we know, the better we feel about ourselves. Some children with brain dysfunction won't try to learn new things because they fear they will make mistakes. Just because they may find it hard to learn *some* things, they think they cannot learn *anything*. Just because they make many mistakes when trying to learn *certain things*, they think that they will make many mistakes with *everything*. As a result they don't learn many things they easily could have learned to do well. If they had not been so scared of mistakes, they would have learned the new things and then felt much better about themselves.

This girl had a lot of trouble learning to read.

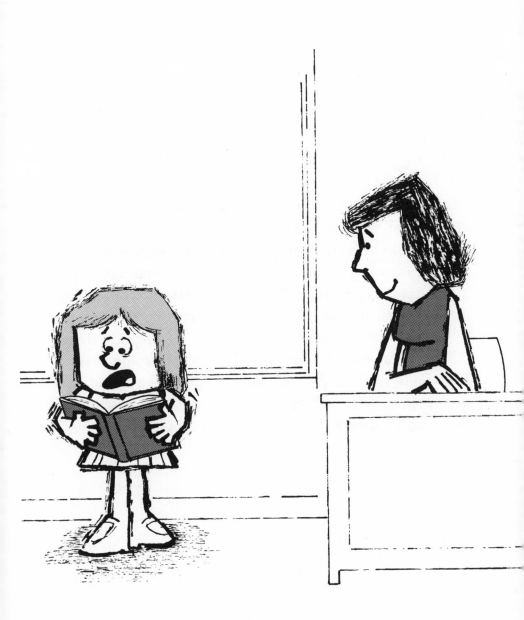

Just because she made a lot of mistakes when she read, she thought she would not be good in anything she tried to learn. She was afraid to try to learn to swim because she thought she would make many mistakes at swimming as well.

Actually she would have been a very good swimmer if she had tried to learn. Her brain dysfunction did not give her any trouble in swimming—only in reading. Of course, she would have made some mistakes while learning to swim. Everybody does. If she had tried to learn, she would have been able to swim well; and then she would have felt much better about herself. It's too bad she didn't try.

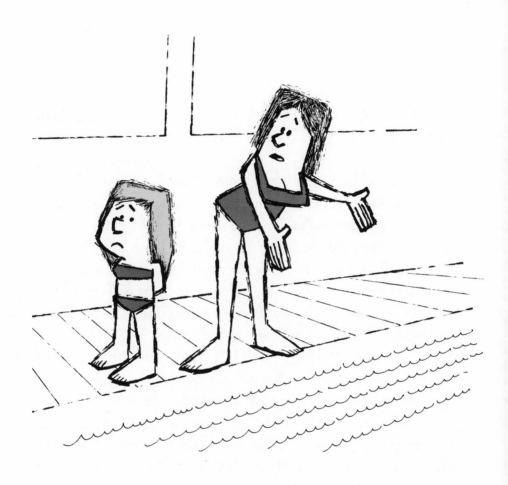

USING BRAIN DYSFUNCTION AS AN EXCUSE FOR GETTING OUT OF DOING WHAT YOU REALLY CAN

Some children with brain dysfunction try to use their problems as an excuse for not doing the things they should.

When this boy's mother asked him to clean up the leaves in the yard, he said, "I can't do it because I've got brain dysfunction." His mother answered, "You may have some trouble in school, but there's no reason why you can't do jobs around the house as well as anyone else. Now you get right out there and clean up the leaves."

Although the boy still didn't want to do the job, a part of him was pleased that his mother thought he could do the jobs around the house as well as anyone else.

Children with brain dysfunction feel good about themselves when they do the jobs their brothers and sisters do. They feel bad about themselves when they try to use their brain dysfunction as an excuse for not doing the jobs they're supposed to do.

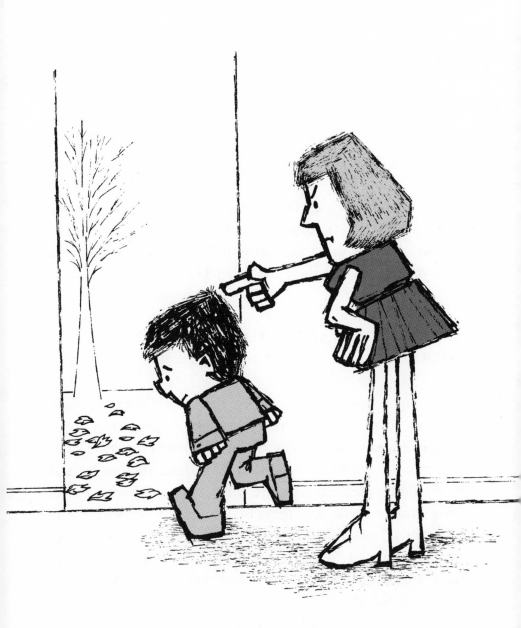

SEEING A THERAPIST

There are some children who get so upset about their brain dysfunction that they need help from a special kind of person called a therapist. Some therapists are psychiatrists or psychologists, but there are other kinds as well.

YOU'RE NOT CRAZY IF YOU HAVE TO SEE A THERAPIST

Some boys and girls think that only "crazy" people have to go to psychiatrists or other types of therapists. If such children then have to see one themselves, they're very ashamed of it, and they feel very bad about themselves and think that something terrible must be wrong with them. Most children who see therapists don't look or behave any differently from other people. They're children who have special problems in a few parts of their lives but who do quite well in most things. Not everything is wrong with them, just a few things.

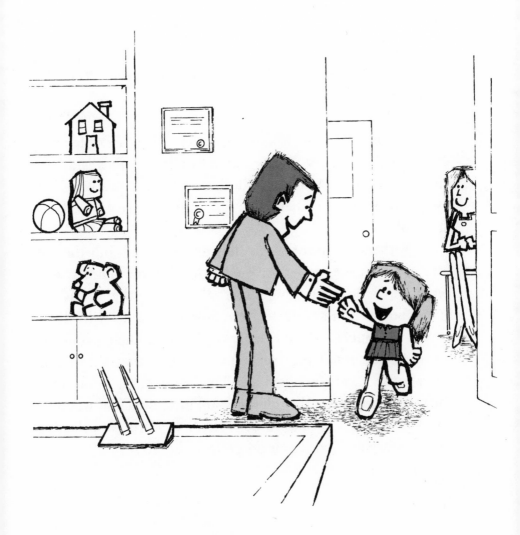

THERE'S NOTHING TO BE ASHAMED OF IF YOU HAVE TO SEE A THERAPIST

Some children who think that it's a terrible and shameful thing to see a therapist refuse to go. This is a bad mistake because then they continue to have problems. If they had gone to a therapist, they might have cleared up many of them.

Others go even though they are ashamed, but they're very careful never to let anyone know they do. They try to keep the whole thing a big secret. They think that if anyone knew, he wouldn't want to have anything to do with them any more. Such children don't realize that their problems are only one small part of themselves and that the rest is often quite good and healthy. They also don't know that the main thing that other children are interested in is whether you are friendly and fun to be with. If you are, they'll want to be with you even if you do go to a therapist.

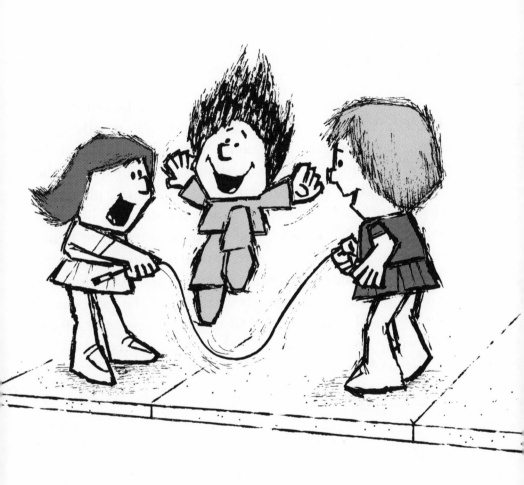

173

WHAT THERAPISTS DO

Let me tell you a little about what therapists do. Although some are doctors, they do not usually give examinations or shots. At times they give pills to help children become less nervous, jumpy, and fussy. At the therapists' office, children usually draw pictures, play with dolls, puppets, and other games, and tell stories. Therapists like to hear about dreams, because dreams tell them something about the problems that are deep inside you, which you may not know too much about. Therapists also talk with children and parents about many of the problems I have discussed in this book. All of these things can help a child worry less and feel better about his troubles.

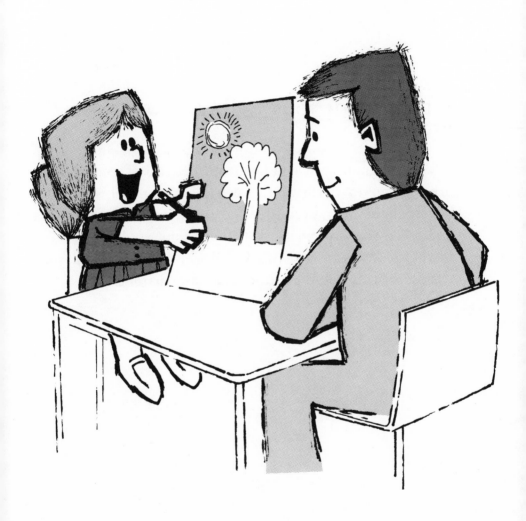

TALKING WITH YOUR PARENTS ABOUT YOUR PROBLEMS

Although most children with brain dysfunction don't need to go to a therapist, they all could feel somewhat better about their problems if they talked to their parents and asked them questions. Whether or not you're going to a therapist, I'm sure you will feel better about some of your troubles if you talk them over with your parents.

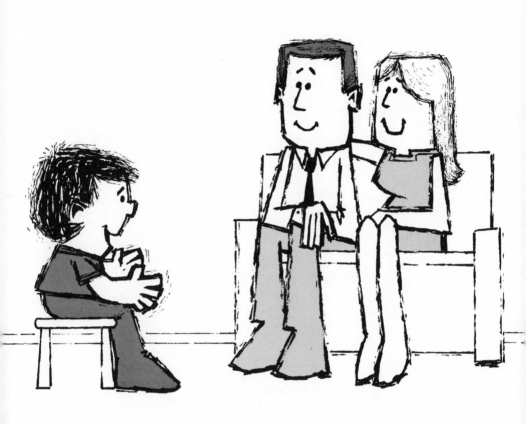

Important Things to Remember

Before I end this book, I would like to repeat a few of the things I have said, to be sure you understand some very important facts.

(1) Everybody has some weaknesses—no one is perfect.

(2) Even when a child has brain dysfunction, most of his brain is still all right.

(3) Just because one or a few parts of your brain are not working well doesn't mean that you are poor in everything. Most of your brain is still perfectly fine, and you can learn to do many things that can help you be happy and useful.

(4) Most boys and girls with minimal brain dysfunction are not retarded, and some are very bright.

(5)   Even without special treatment, many children with brain dysfunction get better and better as they get older, and they catch up to other children.

(6)   Besides treatment from a therapist, there are many other things, such as special classes and special home teaching programs, that can be helpful to the child with brain dysfunction.

(7)   No one can tell in advance what will happen to you in the future. Each test shows you how much better you have gotten since the last test. The tests cannot tell about your future. If you work hard there is a better chance that you will do better in the future.

I have told you many things about boys and girls with minimal brain dysfunction. It is very hard to understand all of these things at once. Read again those parts you do not understand, and ask your parents or therapist to explain to you the things that are still not clear.

Remember!

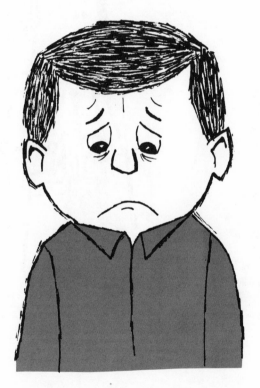

If you are worried about something . . .

. . . talk to your parents . . .

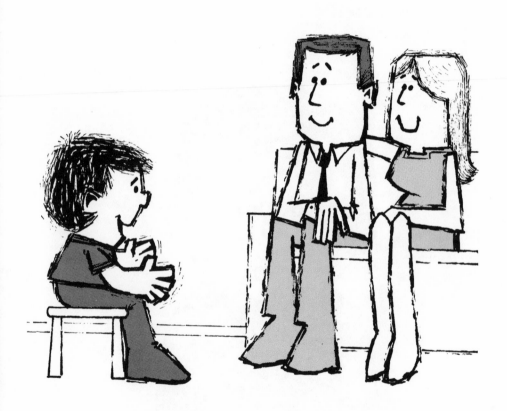

... or therapist, or teacher, about your worries and ask them questions.

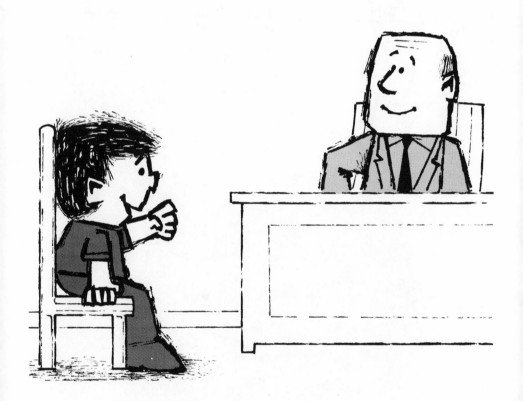

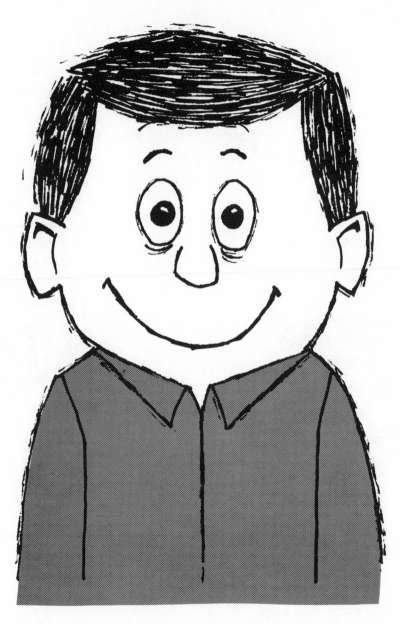

If you do this, I am sure you will feel better about your problems.

Epilogue

I wrote this book because I wished that children with brain dysfunction would read it and that they would then feel better about their troubles. I hope that my wish has come true.

DATE DUE			